As a survivor of leptospirosis, heart attack, hypertension, attempted suicide, type-2 diabetes, peripheral neuropathy, stroke, cardiovascular disease, kidney disease, stage-4 prostate cancer and skin cancer, Robert McAnderson is living proof that, with hope, anything is possible.

In the last three years, Robert has shed over 40 kilograms, achieved diabetic remission, restored kidney function after 20 years, and eliminated eleven prescription medications.

This book would not have been possible were it not for the love and support of my beautiful wife, Jacqui, and the love and support of our three daughters, Courtney, Taylor and Paige.

Jacqui used the words "Fear and Anger" to describe the impact my health issues had on our married life – she lived in fear for 30 years that I would die and she would be left a widow and Anger; she was angry with me because I didn't care enough about her and our daughters to do whatever was required to live a better quality of life and ensure our marriage was robust and healthy.

Jacqui, I cannot undo the damage I have done to you and our daughters but I hope that by sharing this story I may be able to prevent other men, husbands and fathers from making the same mistakes.

Dr. Sarah Barrand B.Med Dip FP, FRACGP
Sarah considers health issues from a holistic approach and has particular interests in supporting patients with weight loss and encouraging a healthy diet and lifestyle through evidence-based techniques. Sarah formed a strong therapeutic bond with Robert over many years and has been instrumental in helping him recover his health.

Robert McAnderson

LIFE IS A GIFT; HEALTH IS A CHOICE, CHOICES HAVE CONSEQUENCES

AUSTIN MACAULEY PUBLISHERS®

LONDON · CAMBRIDGE · NEW YORK · SHARJAH

A CIP catalogue record for this title is available from the British Library.

ISBN 9781035849062 (Paperback)
ISBN 9781035849079 (ePub e-book)

www.austinmacauley.com

First Published 2024
Austin Macauley Publishers Ltd®
1 Canada Square
Canary Wharf
London
E14 5AA

Table of Contents

Foreword   15

Driving Ambition Behind This Book   16

Fundamental Truth About Health   18

Choices   20

Choices Have Consequences   21

Reactive vs Active   22

Heal your Body—Heal your Mind   23

Your Health is Like the Air in a Tyre   26

Chapter: 1 My Health Journey   31

Was This My Legacy   *38*

Photo Album Reflections   *38*

1984: The Start   *39*

1989: Leptospirosis   *40*

1996: Heart Attack   *41*

1998: Hypertension (High Blood Pressure)   *43*

2001: Acute Respiratory Distress   *44*

2004: Sleep Apnoea   *45*

2014: Attempted Suicide   *46*

2014: Planned Suicide   *48*

2015: Diabetes   *49*

2015: Peripheral Neuropathy 51

2018: Stroke 53

2019: Collapse Lung Pneumonia 55

2021: Enlarged Prostate 55

2021: Cardiovascular Disease 57

2022: Kidney Disease 58

2022: Prostate Cancer 58

Summary **71**

Chapter: 2 Life is a Gift **72**

What Determines a Person's Health 75

Does Health Determine Fitness or Fitness Health 76

What's Next 77

Nature or Nurture 77

Pregnancy 78

Summary **84**

Chapter: 3 Health is a Choice **85**

Global Statistics on Obesity 86

Health Risks Linked to Excess Weight and Obesity 88

Heart Attack 89

High Blood Pressure 91

High LDL Cholesterol, Low HDL Cholesterol, High Levels
of Triglycerides 93

Stroke 96

Gallbladder Disease 98

Osteoarthritis 103

Sleep Apnea 104

Cancers 105

Low Quality of Life 105

Mental Illness (Depression) 105

Body Pain and Difficulty with Physical Functioning   *106*

Obesity   *107*

Waist Circumference   *107*

Kidney Disease   *108*

Prostate Cancer   *109*

Summary   **115**

Chapter: 4 Choices Have Consequences   **116**

Medical Conditions That Cause Weight Gain   *117*

Health Effects of Being Overweight or Obese   *117*

Three Elements of Sugar   *119*

Summary   **125**

Chapter: 5 My Why   **128**

My WHY   *130*

Chapter 6 After the Dash   **131**

Knowledge and Wisdom   *131*

Accept Your Fate   *135*

Extend Your Life   *137*

The Choice is Yours   *139*

Summary   **143**

Chapter: 7 Reclaim Your Health   **144**

Retrain Your Mind   *144*

What You Put in Your Stomach   *147*

Physical Activity and Exercise   *148*

Physical Fitness   *150*

Cardiovascular Fitness   *151*

Summary   **152**

Chapter: 8 Soil Degradation   **153**

Examples of Soil Degradation　　155

Declining Nutrient Composition　　156

The Cause of Declining Nutrient Composition　　158

Common Missing Nutrients in Depleted Soil　　159

GMO Foods　　159

Summary　　161

Chapter: 9 Ground and Surface Water Degradation　　162

Water Contaminations　　162

From the Reservoir to the Tap　　163

Water Contamination and Required Treatments　　164

Water Ratios in the Human Body　　165

Summary　　166

Chapter: 10 Nutrition　　167

Food; Quality; Nutrition; Balance　　168

Sugars　　168

Starches　　169

Fibre　　169

Saturated Fats　　170

Unsaturated Fats　　170

Monounsaturated Fats　　170

Polyunsaturated Fats　　170

Sugar　　171

Sugar Substitutes　　171

Junk Food　　172

A Balanced Diet　　173

Summary　　174

Chapter: 11 Supplementation　　177

Probiotic　　177

Omega-3   *178*

Multi-Vitamin   *178*

Cal-Mag D   *178*

Siberian Ginseng and Ginkgo Biloba   *179*

Concentrated Fruits and Vegetables   *180*

Vitamin C Plus   *180*

Glucosamine HCl with Boswellia   *180*

CoQ10   *181*

Magnesium   *181*

Summary   **183**

Chapter: 12 Weight Management   **186**

Choices It's All About Choices   *186*

Basic Regulation of Eating and Body Weight   *187*

Weight   *187*

BMI   *187*

Fat   *188*

Visceral Fat   *188*

Body Age   *188*

Muscle Mass   *189*

Overweight and Obesity   *189*

Healthy Weight Management   *191*

Summary   **192**

Chapter: 13 Mental Health   **194**

Young Adults and Mental Health   *195*

Stigma Associated with Mental Health   *196*

Medication   *197*

Psychological Theories   *198*

Getting Help   *199*

Mental Health Professionals   *199*

Summary   **201**

Chapter: 14 Stress Management   **202**

Types of Stress   *203*

Effects of Stress on the Body   *204*

Summary   **207**

Chapter: 15 Environmental Health   **209**

Ecosystems   *209*

Summary   **213**

Chapter: 16 Long Life or Quality Life   **214**

People are Living Longer   *214*

Unhealthy Aging   *215*

Managing the Aging Process   *215*

Summary   **217**

Chapter: 17 Wellness   **220**

DOSE (Dopamine, Oxytocin, Serotonin, Endorphins)   *220*

Time Changes Everything   *221*

Wellness Influence   *222*

Maintaining Wellness   *223*

Summary   **224**

Chapter: 18 Why Most Diets Don't Work   **226**

Do Diets Work is the Big Question   *226*

Why Don't Diets Work   *230*

One That Does Work   *230*

Weight Loss Goal   *231*

Health Over Diet Works Every Time   *231*

How Did I Allow It to Get This Bad   *231*

What You Do is Who You Are   *232*

Summary   **233**

Chapter: 19 Functional Medicine   **236**

Defence and Repair Node   *236*

Energy Node   *237*

Biotransformation and Elimination Node   *237*

Transport Node   *237*

Communication Node   *238*

Structural Integrity Node   *238*

Assimilation Node   *238*

Summary   **239**

Nutrition and Diet Counselling   **240**

Bibliography   **241**

Index   **243**

Foreword

As we prioritise our health, it's important to recognise the impact of our lifestyle choices on those we love. Robert's story is a powerful reminder of this. While he has made incredible progress in reclaiming his health, the consequences of his past choices have caused significant pain and anguish for his family.

As the head of his household, Robert failed to be the man his wife thought she married and the father his daughters expected and hoped he would be. For 30 years, his family lived in fear that he would die while also feeling angry that he didn't seem to care enough to fight for his health.

But Robert's story is also one of hope. By changing his lifestyle, he has made remarkable progress in his physical and mental health. His passion for openly sharing his psychological and physical struggles is evident in the title of his book and the image of the phoenix rising from the ashes on the cover.

So, if you're looking for a magical solution to your health, you may be disappointed. But if you're open to making lifestyle changes, Robert's story is a powerful reminder that there's always hope. Just remember that your health choices have the potential to impact those you love in ways you couldn't imagine.

Driving Ambition Behind This Book

I am not a remarkable man, but I have been told by many that my health journey, indeed my story, is impressive in that I have survived a heart attack, stroke, kidney disease, cancer, and numerous other health issues that brought me close to death on three occasions and severely damaged my relationship with my wife and daughters.

By that statement, I do not imply that Jacqui and my daughters don't love me or that our relationship is fractured, but the relationship is not what it could have been if I had lived a healthy life and not one plagued by severe health issues. The truth is, I let them down constantly, placing them in situations where my medical conditions caused them untold stress and fear that my health would ultimately fail. This unnecessary burden became even more apparent in recent years when I reversed my type-2 diabetes, high blood pressure, and kidney disease and survived stage-4 cancer. Candidly, it begged the question, if I could do this at seventy-two, why did I not care enough about them to fight harder for my health when I was younger?

My story is simple, and it's shared by numerous other men who, as I did, live in denial that their health is an issue and that they need to take corrective actions or face the consequences of the poor lifestyle choices they make every day.

The following image says it all when it comes to our choices. We are always looking for a quick fix instead of a real solution.

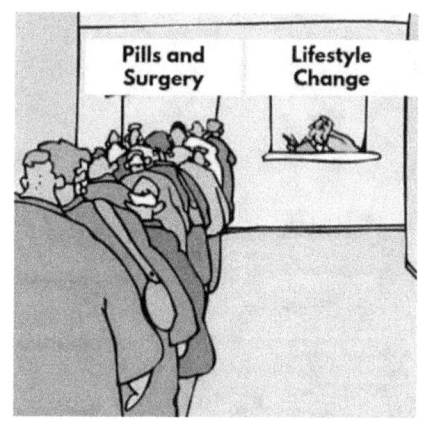

I hope this book and my efforts on social media will encourage men and women of all ages to believe it's possible to reverse medical conditions and reclaim their health. Making lifestyle changes while reducing the use and reliance on prescription medications will deliver results, while surgical interventions must be considered as the last option.

Health can no longer be taken for granted, and unless we change our lifestyle habits and take steps to improve our health, a day and time will come when that health fails, just like it failed me.

Fundamental Truth About Health

Health is like the level of air pressure in a tyre. The first impression is that the average tyre looks fully inflated, but we don't know the actual pressure without measuring it. We assume the pressure will carry us the distance we need to travel and deliver optimal performance.

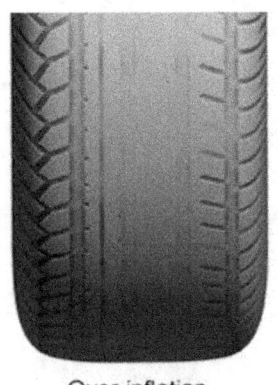 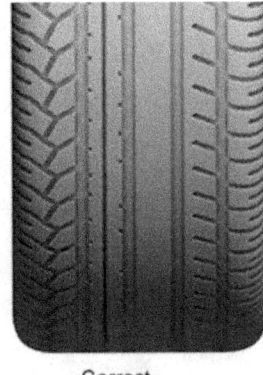

Over-inflation   Correct

Maintaining correct tyre pressure helps keep you (and other road users) safe, improve vehicle performance, decrease fuel costs, and ensure you get the most life out of your tyres. Translated, you will live a healthy lifestyle that will protect and keep your family safe and ensure you live the quality of life many aspire to achieve.

Conversely, an over-inflated tyre can look normal to the average observer, given that wear and tear are not easily seen or corrected. Performance appears normal, but if uncorrected, an over-inflated tyre can unexpectedly fail and endanger the lives of others. Everything seems normal, and slight drops in stamina and performance are almost unnoticeable. Your quality of lifestyle seems consistent, but your health will inevitably fail due to your inability to see the changes in your health over time.

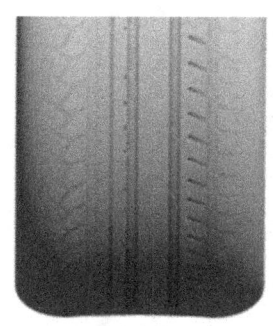

Under-inflation

An under-inflated tyre is easily identified because abnormal wear factors are apparent. At the same time, drop-offs in performance become noticeable, particularly when changes in the weather draw your attention to a loss in traction and an inability to control the vehicle in complex driving situations.

We take health for granted, like the tyre pressure on our car's tyres. Performance drops are hardly noticed, and when they are, we quickly dismiss them, believing you are having an off day. Until you hit a pothole or extreme weather conditions, draw our attention to the problem. For me, those extreme conditions were a heart attack and, several years later, a stroke.

Low air pressure causes extensive wear and is the number one cause of tyre blowouts and failures.

The human body is no different from that tyre; as it ages, it is more prone to performance issues. Our journey through life is not always on expressways and perfect roads but occasionally over broken and weather surfaces, across flooded creeks and rough, damaged surfaces. At this time, those blowouts and failures are the equivalents of heart attacks and strokes.

Your choice. You can wait until the tyre is flat or make the decision to check your tyre pressure frequently, ensuring you achieve the greatest return on investment you will ever make, including your health.

Choices

In the movie *Sliding Doors*, Helen (Gwyneth Paltrow), a London ad executive, is fired from her job and rushes out to catch a train; two scenarios occur. In one, she gets on the train and comes home to find her boyfriend, Gerry (John Lynch), in bed with another woman; Helen dumps Gerry, finds a new man and gradually improves her life. In the second, she becomes suspicious of Gerry's fidelity and grows miserable, misses the train, arrives after the woman has left, and lives a life with an unfaithful husband.

Choices Have Consequences

My wife, Jacqui, recently asked me why it took thirty years to realise that if I didn't change my lifestyle, exercise, and eating habits, I would die earlier than I would have liked. This question left me deep in thought for an unusually long time, struggling to articulate an acceptable response and prompting Jacqui to ask me if I heard her or was avoiding the question.

Even now, reflecting on that question spirals me into confusion and anxiety that is hard to explain. I didn't make the choices I did, knowing those would lead to a life-threatening situation and yet I have to ask myself how many warning signs a person needs before they see the light and take action.

The answer to that question is why I decided to write this book and actively engage in a social media campaign focusing on 'Reclaim Your Health'. I believe people, myself included, get caught up living life with all of its distractions rather than enjoying the quality of the life we could live if only we dared to do whatever it takes to realise that quality.

It's what I would call a reactive lifestyle.

Reactive vs Active

Allowing the pressures of life to consume our time, energy, and life force is a fact few people will deny. Technological advances have found ways to extend our working hours while at the same time changing our work from physical to more sedimentary activity with increased screen-based activities.

The challenge many of us face is that we don't believe we have a health issue; I certainly didn't, so dedicating time and effort to exercise is not the priority, and time availability becomes the excuse.

Had I decided to actively engage in any activity that would have improved my health and avoided the medical dramas that caused me such difficulties, I wonder what my life would look like today.

Instead, I was forced to reactively take steps to recover my health, hoping these activities would reverse some medical conditions and improve my health.

It's your choice; you can actively engage in any process that maintains or improves your health or wait until a health issue forces you to make reactive changes to your lifestyle.

The human body possesses an enormous, astonishing, and persistent capacity to heal itself. Every second we're alive, the cells in our bodies endlessly work to bring us back to a natural state of homeostasis or equilibrium. When we turn to medicines or physical manipulations to heal our bodies, it's for one reason: we have ignored the body's warning signals or neglected our health by depriving our bodies of the basic requirements to keep us healthy.

When a large number of cells are killed, the surrounding cells replicate to make new cells, thereby quickly replacing the damaged cells. Cells can heal themselves while new cells replace permanently damaged or destroyed cells. Each cell is a dynamic, living unit constantly monitoring and adjusting its processes, working to restore itself according to the original DNA code it was created with and maintaining balance within the body.

Heal your Body—Heal your Mind

Regardless of your current health, I believe healing yourself by being positive, optimistic and focused is possible. With a positive mental attitude, physiological changes in your body strengthen your immune system, decrease pain, and relieve stress.

The changes begin when your subconscious mind picks up the new belief system, eliminating and replacing some habits. Once established, these new neural pathways will lead us towards the health we want and need.

To better understand what I am saying, you need to understand my life before I woke up at seventy-two to realise that all my lifestyle "Choices had Consequences."

Over the past thirty-two years, my health has been in decline. While you might say that is normal, it's called the ageing process; I am talking about an accelerated decline caused by my repeated failure to acknowledge and correct the lifestyle habits that were the root cause of my health issues.

I have relied on doctors and specialists to remove organs, or repair damaged body parts surgically, treated me symptomatically, and prescribed medications that have managed my declining conditions rather than offering solutions that would address the cause of these medical conditions.

My health was adversely affected in 1989 when I contracted Leptospirosis, which damaged my kidneys, and that was the beginning of my hypertension issues, with which I am still struggling.

While Leptospirosis may have been a starting point, you must understand that my health declined over thirty years because I thought I was indestructible and refused to make the necessary changes to my lifestyle. Being overweight for most of my life was the symptom, not the cause, of my declining health; my indulgencies in food and alcohol and a lack of desire to maintain a fitness level to balance these indulgences were my issues.

I was unwilling to change these lifestyle habits and failed to recognise the impact on my health.

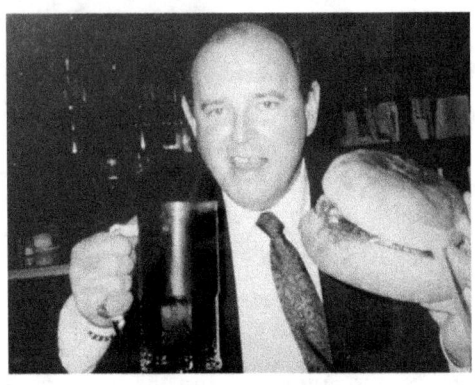

With age comes wisdom, and while that wisdom has helped me identify the lifestyle habits that consumed my health, it has also made me realise that I will not have enough time to reverse the damage I have done to my health.

In 2022, I had four cancer surgeries, two melanomas, one on my cheek and another on my shin, three early-stage cancers in my bowel and one Type 4, Gleeson 8 Prostate Cancer that had already started to metastasise.

While my skin cancers can be attributed to the numerous hours I spent in the sun without sunblock, medical research has confirmed that both bowel and prostate cancer are significantly linked to obesity, poor diet and alcohol. These lifestyle choices are related to the increasing number of cancer cases and deaths, while smoking is still the most significant cause of cancer and cancer deaths.

The combination of excess body weight, alcohol intake, poor diet, and physical inactivity accounted for the highest proportion of all cancer cases in women. It was second only to tobacco smoking in men.

These four combined risk factors also accounted for the second-highest proportion of cancer deaths in both men and women.

Diet was significant for colon cancer, with red and processed meat consumption accounting for 5.4% and 8.2% of colorectal cancers, respectively. Low dietary fibre accounted for 10.3% of colorectal cancer cases, and low dietary calcium accounted for 4.9%.

I assembled a collection of my blood test results to prepare for writing this book. While doing so, I realised that the damage done to my kidneys by leptospirosis placed me in the Stage 3b Kidney Disease category with a life expectancy of eight years.

In chapter one, under the sub-heading "Understanding Blood Test Results", I have included a history of my blood test results, which shows my kidneys' declining functionality. In addition, it also highlights that I have been able to reverse the functionality of my kidneys. Still, it's important to note that the damage to my kidneys is irreversible.

There are many reasons why writing this book has become such a passionate venture for me. Still, their greatest desire is to help other indestructible men realise wisdom can be found before stupidity becomes a consequence we cannot reverse.

Your Health is Like the Air in a Tyre

It's not until the air pressure drops to a point where performance becomes an issue that the consequences become apparent, ignoring that loss in tyre pressure will result in a complete failure.

As you will see in the coming chapters, I missed all the warning signs and, as a result, was under the care of six specialists, all of whom kept telling me I needed to change my lifestyle and habits.

Habits are the most challenging things to change, and the older you are, the more entrenched those habits become.

In September 2020, I reached a point where my wife reconciled herself to the fact that she would be a widow and end up living with her mother.

I was 137.2 kilograms, had a BMI of 36, suffered from chronically high blood pressure and was a type-2 diabetic. With diabetes came a lovely condition called peripheral neuropathy, resulting in severe nerve pain in my legs.

Candidly, it was time to change the flat tyre or learn to accept the consequences of my abysmal health choices.

I took photographs of myself (see Image 1) and put them into the Notes section of my iPhone, along with measurements of my chest, waist and hips. At this point, I started my journey to reclaim my health.

I did not set out to become the example, but I understood that at seventy-two, it was possible to change my habits and reverse many of the medical conditions that plagued my life. I did not know then that I would commit to recording sixty-second posts on Instagram, creating a website or writing this book dedicated to documenting my health journey. Along the way, I had people ask me how much weight I had lost, and the answer I gave them was the story of my health journey, and from telling that story, I developed a passion for reclaiming my health and others who my story could influence.

My passion for poking, prodding, encouraging, tempting or persuading anyone who would listen to me that unless they accepted, their health was a choice and those choices have consequences, the quality of their life would never be improved.

Along the way, I concluded that despite my health issues, I wanted to live a longer life and a better quality of life.

Having dropped 34 kilograms in weight, reduced my BMI to 25, cured my Type-2 diabetes, reduced my blood pressure medication by 50% and eliminated my pain medication along with fourteen other prescription medications, I was ready for a new challenge.

Be careful what you ask for because sometimes you may not like what you receive.

I had just finished the second draft of this book when my next challenge was revealed.

After three weeks of waiting for MRI, Biopsy and PET scan results, Stage-4, Gleason-8 Prostate Cancer, and surgery became my next challenge. I don't think I will ever forget how the doctor's staff looked at me on the day of revelation. It was like they knew the results and what the doctor would tell me, and sympathetically, they were reaching out to me in a non-verbal way, telling me they were sorry. Then, after walking into the doctor's room, exchanging pleasantries and being told a joke before the bad news was further confirmed.

On reflection, I think both Jacqui and I were half expecting the results of the biopsy to be bad while hoping the results of the tests would ultimately be a little better than stage-4 cancer.

I don't think we spoke to each other as we walked to the lifts after leaving the doctor's surgery. On our walk back to the car, Jacqui commented, 'While the cancer was outside the prostate, the PET scan results confirmed cancer had not metastasised to other parts of my body was a good outcome,' followed by, 'we will work through this; it's all going to be OK.'

Finally, I turned to Jacqui and said, it's just another chapter in the book.

This journey started as a chronicle of my poor health choices and their related consequences, and I hope that finishing the book may inspire others, helping them reclaim their health. I hope people who read my story will understand that if a seventy-two-year-old man with my medical history could lose weight and reverse the medical issues that have plagued his health for thirty years, others could do the same regardless of age.

Using my extensive social media following on Twitter and Instagram, I decided to promote the need for people to look more acutely at their health and lifestyle habits and make changes where needed. Short sixty-second videos and text messages encourage people to believe that changing habits can change the quality of their health.

Still, I am committed to reclaiming my health, and with changes to a person's lifestyle, anyone who genuinely wants the same outcome can achieve what I have done.

It all started with getting up off the couch, feeding my brain with positive messages, my stomach with quality food in the right combination of proteins, carbohydrates and fats, and committing to walking every morning before breakfast, rail hail or shine.

As a result, I lost weight, and my body started to repair itself.

For details on these changes, see the historical blood test result on page 70.

Enjoy the book, and if I can leave you with one thought, it would be this.

Life is a Gift; Health is a Choice, and choices have consequences.
3,153,600,000. How many do you have left?

"It has been said that time heals all wounds. The truth is that time does not heal anything. It merely passes. It is what we do during the passing of time that helps or hinders the healing proce0ss."

– Jay Marshall

Chapter 1
My Health Journey

It is universally believed that men reach their physical peak in their late twenties to early thirties and their cognitive peak in their mid-thirties. But when it comes to a man's health, I believe all men think they are bulletproof and, on many occasions, refuse to accept the obvious even when their doctors present the facts.

I am not sure what category I fell into, given that from age thirty-five, it took me thirty-seven years and three months to accept all the warning signs about my failing health before I took any corrective action.

On reflection, I would have to call it stupidity, given my history and obstinate refusal to heed the warning signs.

On numerous occasions, Jacqui has asked me what caused me to decide to reclaim my health, and on every occasion, I responded by saying I don't know.

On Sunday, 5 March 2023, when Jacqui asked me again, I finally knew the answer. We were sitting in a café having our regular Sunday morning breakfast, and on the table in front of me was my phone. In it were all the text messages I had written detailing my feelings, my depression, my struggles, and yes, even my final goodbyes.

In the following few pages, I will share some text messages I recorded on my phone. They are personal and were written to my wife and children by a man who finally concluded that his life was approaching an end.

On this same day, I decided to include some of these personal messages in this book because I realised that when I started writing them, I started fighting for my life, which was the beginning of my journey to recover my health.

6 August 2019

I had a great day yesterday with you visiting the cemeteries to gather competitive information about their operations. What a joy it was to watch your face light up with that unbelievable smile as we joked about telling Frank what we had said to the staff at the cemetery.

Our Cover Story

We were researching the cost of Mausoleums for our close friend, "Frank", who was close to passing.

I love you so very much it's hard to describe in words.
Spending the day with you was an unexpected reward this week for me.

7 August 2019

Intense pain in one toe of my left foot last night, and the painkillers did nothing. I woke at 2:00, went back to sleep at 5:00, and slept till 7:00.

Sleep quality is 60%, with acute pain and thoughts about cutting off my toe. The only trouble I fear is that I am unsure which toe to cut off, given that my feet and legs are numb from the nerve damage caused by diabetes.

I am feeling very depressed; the pain has been constant for over seventeen hours, and I don't think it will ease anytime soon.

Without my promise to you and the kids that I would not attempt suicide again, I think the dark thoughts that haunt me would have their way with me.

21 August 2019

Currently sitting in the park trying to force myself to get up, walk home back into our house, knowing how much you love me and get on with my life.

I never deserved the love you have shown me, but I think that is because I didn't know what love was until I met you.

Ironic because at 11:30, halfway through writing this note, you just called me to see how I was.

My journey is not over, and I will push through this dark space precisely because of your love for me.

December 2019

To put this message in a time context, we are both sitting in our favourite spot on the stern of the Carnival Spirit on Thursday, 4 December, having just finished breakfast.

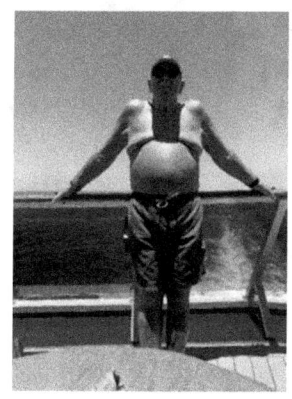

We joked about me getting old and how you would kick me to the kerb and start looking for a replacement because I haven't looked after myself.

Thank you for all the love you showed me during our time together and the sacrifices you made for me.

Katoomba was a dark time for you when I planned my second suicide, but while you struggled on multiple fronts during that period, your love was the beacon that allowed me to find my way home.

December 2019

I have partially collapsed left lung and pneumonia, just sitting at home waiting for the love of my life to come home.

After spending eleven days and nights with you on the cruise, it is strange to sit here at home waiting for you to get home from work. I want you to know that I love you and think of you every spare moment of my day.

So, if this condition takes a turn for the worse and I end up in hospital with pneumonia, I want you to know that I love you, and I'm sorry our cruise holiday ended so poorly.

January 2020

Sitting on the train thinking about our life together, what we have created, won, lost and shared. Quite honestly, I would not trade a single moment.

My wish from the moment I saw you walking down the aisle on the arm of your father was that I would spend my life in the company of that beautiful woman.

It may come as a surprise, but I still have that vision firmly embedded in my mind, and when I look at you, I still see that beautiful woman.

Others see a strength in you, but you don't believe it exists. I promise you this; the time is coming when it will burst out of you like an alien in the movie.

At that time, take a deep breath, surrender to your inner strength, trust your instincts, and let the juices flow.

You have been on a journey of self-discovery, and all the pieces of your life puzzle are just about ready to reveal the big picture.

I have been writing these notes for you as an encouragement and to ensure you have something from me to remember me.

Photos are one thing, my paintings another, but the one thing about me you were attracted to from the beginning was my brain, so writing these notes to you is how I can still reach out to you when I am no longer here.

So when you hear the tap tap tap in the middle of the night, know I am still with you, if only in spirit.

21 March 2020

I was sitting here watching TV with you after a restless night with much pain. I woke up several times troubled by what felt like joint pain and concerned I may have covid-19. It occurred to me that, given my medical history, I would be isolated in a hospital and not have a chance to say goodbye.

11 July 2020

To my three beautiful daughters

I sit at home alone; Paige is at work tonight, Taylor is out with Gui, Courtney is with Josh, and Jacqui is at a weight loss coaching meeting. I ordered pizza, reflected on my role as a father, and wondered how many things I would have done differently had I the chance to do it all over again.

I genuinely love each of you and am so very proud of who you are and what you are doing with your lives—all beautiful young women with a strength most would envy.

My inability to control my anger was an issue for me, and I know each of you experienced this first-hand, and I apologise.

I hope you will never forget to think of me lovingly because I believe each of you to be my best work of art.

Love always
Your Father

14 August 2020

I just walked up to the Ponds and bought bread and soup for lunch, plus a coffee to sit and reflect before walking home.

I have had a wonderful life being with you, and I have changed so much because of the unconditional love you have shown me.

I sometimes wonder where I would be and what I would be doing if not for you.

The line I used way back in time that encouraged you to relax and go out with me for that first drink and then the dinner at the Three Doors Restaurant to make up for your missing dinner with your parents was somewhat true.

"I am too old for you".

In some way, I have cheated you by not thinking about what our possible lives would look like thirty-plus years ahead.

I apologise for everything you have had to put up with regarding my health and all that you will miss out on because of our age difference and all my numerous health issues.

I hope, in some way, the knowledge of how much I love you makes up for all you have missed.

While I don't think anyone could have loved you more than I do, I am not sure that is adequate compensation for all I stole from you.

Etched indelibly in my mind are four images of you.

1. *The white dress you wore the day you presented AIIMS to my team in the ground floor meeting room of 3M.*
2. *The low-back dress you wore on our first date at the Thee Doors restaurant.*
3. *The day you stole my heart and head in your wedding dress when your father walked you down the aisle.*
4. *On the footsteps of the art gallery and the photo I took of you with that beautiful head of hair swept over your face.*

While thousands more are in my head, these four images constantly come to the front of my mind.

September 2020

#MyWeightLossJourney

Today, I committed to controlling my eating habits when I realised that I always wanted to eat more after eating.

So what is this going to look like going forward?

137.9kg this morning.

Three meals a day, starting with carbs for breakfast, fruit for lunch and a small meal for dinner.

I will commit to 8,000 to 11,000 steps daily and some upper body exercises.

My goal is 105kg and less pain management medicine.

Stomach 133cm

Chest 133cm

Hips 119cm

These legs have given me enough shit, so now I will give them some shit back as I push them, walking long distances every day.

As ridiculous as this sounds, I want to be fit enough to jog building to a point where I can run two kilometres continuously.

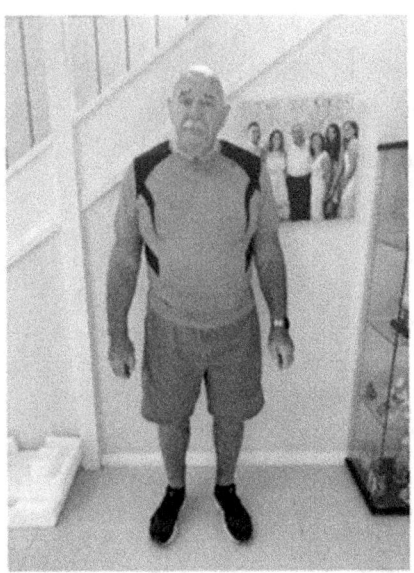 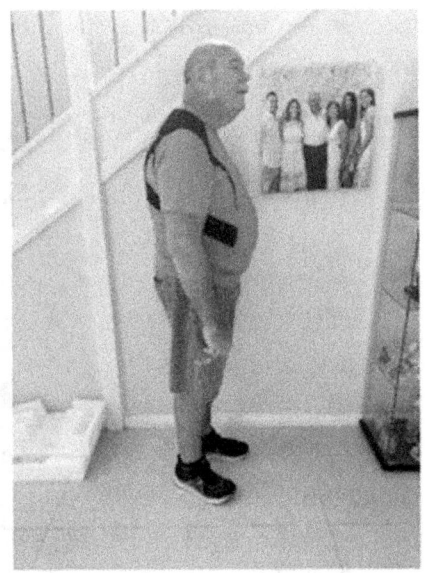

A bit ambitious for my age and condition, but I have always believed in setting significant goals and, even if I fall short, still achieving an outcome far over anything anyone thought was possible.

When I hear the term "Legacy", I think about what I have accumulated that will be passed on to my wife and children after my death. I don't know if your thinking is similar to mine, or maybe it is not something you have thought about.

We are encouraged to make a will to ensure those things we consider valuable are passed onto a family member or someone we know or love instead of being grabbed by the government. The last thing we want to happen is for our legacy to be thrown into consolidated government revenue or claimed by someone who supposedly had a meaningful connection with you at some time in the past.

Is that what best describes the term legacy?

While I found several definitions on the internet and various dictionaries, I thought the following described it best.

"Leaving behind a legacy means making an impact that will last long after you die. It could be financial, with something you create, or through the people you touch while alive".

The good news is that it's never too late to start working on building a legacy that will outlive you, and that is what I committed to doing when I began posting my one-minute video clips about health on Instagram and started writing this book.

For me, it's not about building wealth or that elusive fifteen minutes of fame people talk about; for me, it is all about helping people of all genders and ages realise that if they don't take steps to reclaim their health, their health will let them down in a big way and most probably at the worst possible time.

The book's title summarises my passion for creating this legacy: "Life is a Gift; Health is a Choice, and Choices have Consequences".

I should know that because of my poor health choices and lack of commitment to look after my health, I walk on the consequences of Type-2 diabetes nerve damage caused to my legs daily.

In the opinion of my neurologist, the nerve damage in my legs will ultimately see me confined to a wheelchair.

While this medical condition is just one of several I am dealing with, the most significant damage I have done is not to my body but to my wife's and children's mental health, for I failed to see the damage I was doing to them until my wife Jacqui summed up her feelings about how she felt when I had her record a short video she did for me to post on Instagram.

In that video, she told me the two words that summed up her feelings about my health.

Fear and Anger: fear she lived with for over thirty years that I would die. She would be left alone a widow, and Anger: she was angry with me because I did not care enough about her and our daughters to do whatever was required to live a better quality of life and ensure our marriage was robust and healthy and be the father to our daughters deserved.

Was This My Legacy

Was this really what I wanted to leave for my family, for the wife and daughters that mean the world to me, a memory of a man who didn't care enough about them, didn't love them enough to fight for his life, to be the husband and father they were angry with rather than the one they loved, respected, and admired.

What Was I Thinking?

A legacy that's the word that drives me now; that's the focus I needed; my health journey is no longer a weight loss journey. Instead, it has become the passion that drives me like the mythical ancient bird, the phoenix. I will rise from my sickness, overcome my health obstacles, and stand tall and proud of the legacy I leave behind.

For my legacy is you, you and others who will hear, read and see my message and hopefully be inspired to believe that if a seventy-four-year-old man can do what I have done, overcome my health issues, extend the quality and length of my life and win the love respect and admiration of my wife and daughters and stand tall and proud of all, I have accomplished, *then you can as well.*

If you can't do this for yourself, then I tell you, you need to do it for the people you love and who love you because they don't deserve to live in fear of your death or to be angry with you because you didn't care enough about them to do whatever it takes to reclaim your health.

Photo Album Reflections

Recently, I had the chance to look at some old photo albums, and while it was a great time to reminisce, it also caused me to reflect on my photographs over several years. Unsurprisingly, I carried more weight in most pictures than I should have. The funny thing is that at the time, my health seemed to be OK, perhaps not fantastic, but I was not on any medication and could do most of the things I wanted and needed to do.

Like most young men, I played a couple of sports in winter and a different sport in summer. Being physically fit for both sports was an obvious requirement, so I went to training two nights a week and played on the weekend, while in summer, I swam laps at the local pool and five days a week early in the morning, trained two nights a week and played grade water polo on the weekends.

When I look at images from those years until I reached my early thirties, it is clear I was in reasonable shape, so the big question is, where did it all start to go wrong, and what triggered my weight/health battle?

1984: The Start

I worked as a state sales manager, putting in the hours and pushing myself to do the job better than I had witnessed and experienced as a salesperson. I followed the philosophy, "You earn your salary between 9:00 to 5:00 and your promotion from 5:00 to 9:00". While this approach resulted in promotion to national sales manager a few years later, it came at a cost that I did not realise for almost thirty years.

At the time, I smoked one and a half packets of cigarettes a day and drank over a dozen cups of coffee. It is not hard to see where this approach would lead: long hours, poor eating habits, and over-the-top caffeine and nicotine stimulants.

It was a typical Tuesday; it was my planning day, time to review the specific training I needed to do for each person in my sales team and allocate the time I would spend with each person. I arrived in the office at 6:45, filled the coffee percolator, and sat to have my usual breakfast, coffee and a cigarette. Around 11:00, I stood up to go to the toilet and felt I was going to pass out.

Head spinning and nauseous, I decided I needed to see someone, so I made an appointment with a doctor just up the road, given that I did not have a regular doctor. He asked me several questions: how many hours I worked, what I had for breakfast and lunch, did I smoked or drink coffee, and did I had sugar in my coffee, and if so, how much sugar.

The answer was no, I did not eat breakfast, nor had I eaten any lunch. I had consumed several cups of coffee, each with a spoonful of sugar, and I had smoked over ten cigarettes.

The doctor looked at me and said there was no solid food in my stomach, and a continuous hit of caffeine, nicotine and sugar was pushing my system to its limits. He went on to explain that sugar is as addictive as cocaine, plus my ability to process that quantity of sugar would always be an issue for my pancreas and insulin production. Was it any wonder I was feeling light-headed?

I didn't realise then that this was the beginning of my diabetes.

What Changed: Nothing

1989: Leptospirosis

My first health scare occurred when I was forty-one, on holiday at Goolwa Island in South Australia.

While walking on the rocks by the river's edge, I cut the bottom of my foot and thought absolutely nothing of it; it was such a small cut.

Jacqui and I started our drive back to Sydney the next day, and it became apparent that I had a significant problem. Uncontrollable chills and fever and wrapped in a blanket, we drove straight to Sydney rather than stop at Wagga Wagga overnight as planned.

Five days passed with me unable to hold anything down; even a glass of water went down and came straight back up.

Jacqui called the local doctor, who advised plenty of fluids and Panadol for the headaches and fever after visiting. Jacqui was beside herself, not knowing what to do given that my condition continued deteriorating.

Finally, we decided she needed to call an ambulance, but Jacqui cleaned the unit up a little before she did. Go figure; it has been a story that brought several laughs over dinner tables and in conversations with friends.

The ambulance transported me to Canterbury Bankstown Hospital. Because I was so dehydrated, unshaven, and smelly, and because AIDS was rampant then, I was left on a gurney in the hallway, and no one wanted to touch me. At that point, a doctor walking past me stopped and looked at my admission chart. He asked me several questions and told me he believed I had leptospirosis or, as we came affectionately to call it, Rats Piss Poisoning.

Leptospirosis

Common symptoms of leptospirosis include fever, severe headache, sore muscles, chills, vomiting, and red eyes. Symptoms usually come on suddenly. These symptoms mimic other diseases, such as influenza, and diagnosis is often difficult. People with leptospirosis may have some or all these symptoms. Some people can also develop long-lasting effects following leptospirosis infection.

These include kidney failure, jaundice (yellow colouration of the skin and eyeballs indicating liver disease), and bleeding and respiratory complications. Other complications, including meningitis (inflammation of the brain and spinal cord), can also occur. Most people who develop severe disease require hospitalisation, and severe leptospirosis can sometimes be fatal.

Symptoms usually develop after five to fourteen days following infection, lasting from a few days to three weeks.

How It Spreads

- *Leptospira bacteria usually enter the body through skin cuts or abrasions and occasionally through the mouth, nose, and eye lining.*
- *Infections are usually associated with exposure to water, soil or mud contaminated with the urine from infected animals.*
- *Many different animals can harbour Leptospira bacteria in their kidneys.*
- *Eating contaminated food or drinking contaminated water has occasionally been responsible for transmission.*
- *Leptospirosis is not generally spread from person to person.*

Leptospirosis is transmitted from animals, most commonly rodents. The bacteria are spread to humans through animal urine or water and soil contaminated with animal urine, coming into contact with the eyes, mouth, nose or breaks in the skin.

Treatment involved intense treatment with antibiotics, anti-noisier medication, and hydration while allowing the kidneys to function correctly again.

My kidneys were severely damaged, believed to be the root cause of many of the high blood pressure issues I experienced later in life.

1996: Heart Attack

My second scare occurred when I was forty-eight. At the time, I was working for a company that ran exhibitions in Manly and living in Baulkham Hills; it was a good sixty-minute drive either way.

The job was not high-pressure but I had significant issues with a friend who convinced me to join his company by offering me a small shareholding.

The pressure that day centred around my partner wanting to terminate a staff member and my resistance to the idea, given that I believed they were a solid performer with good potential if allowed to settle into the role.

As I approached Baulkham Hills on my way home that evening, I started to experience chest pain. It grew in intensity to the point that I drove to what was then the Emergency Department of the Baulkham Hills Private Hospital.

Around 5:30 in the afternoon, I was in the intensive care ward hooked up to an ECG machine when the doctor told me they were waiting on the blood test results to determine if I had a heart attack.

At this point, I started to worry about letting Jacqui know where I was and what had happened, but I didn't want to make that call until blood tests confirmed that I had experienced a heart attack.

The blood test result came back around 7:00, confirming an increase in troponin protein in my blood, indicating I had a mild heart attack.

After my doctor confirmed I had experienced a heart attack and was going to admit me to the hospital, I had no choice other than to call Jacqui and tell her where I was and what had happened.

I was lying in bed thinking, "What the hell am I going to say?".

My work hours were irregular, and while I usually arrived home around 7:00, I knew Jacqui would be expecting me home, so I made the call and fumbled through the conversation, explaining that I was not feeling well while driving home and had stopped at the hospital and then just blurted out the rest.

Heart Attack Warning Signs and Symptoms

Recognising the symptoms of a heart attack and calling Triple Zero (000) *could save your life or the life of a loved one. It's crucial that everyone, both male and female, know a heart attack's warning signs and symptoms because early treatment is vital. The longer a blockage is left untreated, the more damage occurs. The most common heart attack warning signs are:*

- *Chest discomfort or pain (angina) can feel like uncomfortable pressure, aching, numbness, squeezing, fullness or pain in your chest. This discomfort can spread to your arms, neck, jaw or back. It can last for several minutes or come and go.*
- *Dizziness, light-headedness, feeling faint or feeling anxious*
- *Nausea, indigestion, vomiting.*
- *Shortness of breath or difficulty breathing, with or without chest discomfort.*
- *Sweating or a cold sweat.*

1998: Hypertension (High Blood Pressure)

My next medical issue resulted from the undiagnosed Sleep Apnoea, with me walking up in a sweat with an exceptionally high blood pressure of 180/120 and my body producing adrenalin trying to shock me into breathing because of a lack of oxygen.

Back to my kidneys with possible links to leptospirosis and high blood pressure. My neighbour, an insurance actuary, had strong connections in the medical fraternity and suggested I get a referral to Dr Nankivell, a nephrologist (kidney specialist). After seeing Dr Nankivell, he ordered a complete change in medication. A few weeks later, I was again in good space, feeling better and denying that any of these issues were causing other complications.

Hypertension

What is Hypertension or High Blood Pressure? It is when your blood pressure increases to unhealthy levels.

Your blood pressure measurement considers how much blood passes through your blood vessels and the amount of resistance the blood meets while pumping.

Narrow arteries increase resistance. The narrower your arteries are, the higher your blood pressure will be. Over the long term, any increase in your blood pressure can cause health issues, including heart disease.

Hypertension is quite common, with one in every four men and one in every five women in Australia suffering from high blood pressure.

Hypertension typically develops over several years. Usually, you don't notice any symptoms. But even without symptoms, high blood pressure can cause damage to your blood vessels and organs, especially the brain, heart, eyes, and kidneys.

Early detection is essential. Regular blood pressure readings help you and your doctor notice any changes. Elevated blood pressure should be checked over a few weeks to see if the results return to normal.

Treatment for hypertension includes both prescription medication and healthy lifestyle changes. If the condition isn't treated, it could lead to health issues, including heart attack and stroke.

What Causes High Blood Pressure

For most adults, there's no identifiable cause of high blood pressure. This type of high blood pressure, called primary (essential) hypertension, tends to develop gradually over many years.

Some people have high blood pressure caused by an underlying condition. This type of high blood pressure, called secondary hypertension, tends to appear suddenly and cause higher blood pressure than primary hypertension. These conditions and medications can lead to secondary hypertension, including:

- *Obstructive sleep apnoea*
- *Kidney disease*
- *Adrenal gland tumours*
- *Thyroid problems*
- *Certain defects you're born with (congenital) in blood vessels*
- *Certain medications, such as birth control pills, cold remedies, decongestants, over-the-counter pain relievers and some prescription drugs*
- *Illegal drugs, such as cocaine and amphetamines*

2001: Acute Respiratory Distress

I remember sitting outside on a beautiful summer night on New Year's Eve and asking Jacqui and my three daughters to think about a New Year's Eve wish for the coming year. One of my daughters wished I would have a year without health issues, and the rest of the girls jumped on that idea, so it was decided I would not get ill or have any more health issues in the next twelve months.

The next day, I was taken to the Emergency Department at Baulkham Hills Private Hospital with a collapsed lung and acute respiratory problems. The doctor who looked after me had no idea what caused this problem so much for New Year's resolutions.

Acute respiratory distress syndrome (ARDS) occurs when fluid builds up in your lungs' tiny, elastic air sacs (alveoli). The fluid keeps your lungs from filling with enough air, which means less oxygen reaches your bloodstream, depriving your organs of the needed oxygen.

2004: Sleep Apnoea

I was driving home with my three daughters in the car when I realised I was driving in a different lane. I fell asleep behind the car's wheel in that nanosecond and drifted into the right-hand lane. I am sure the drivers on all sides believed I had just changed lanes without using my indicators.

That was a wake-up call; I put so many lives at risk while driving on an expressway at over a hundred kilometres an hour, and it shook me to the core.

My regular doctor referred me to Dr Michail, a respiratory physician who organised a sleepover at Westmead Hospital, where my sleep patterns were monitored and recorded.

A person who experiences a Sleep Apnoea episode less than five times a night is considered normal; from five to fifteen denotes mild sleep apnoea, fifteen to thirty is moderate, while a greater than thirty is deemed severe. My score that night was seventy-five.

There are two types of sleep apnoea.

- Obstructive sleep apnoea is the more common form when throat muscles relax.
- Central sleep apnoea occurs when your brain doesn't signal the muscles you use to breathe appropriately.

I don't do anything by halves. Of course, I have the second form, where the brain doesn't send proper signals to the muscles that control breathing.

My scorecard from the sleepover night at Westmead Hospital indicated a greater than 30 AHI, considered severe, while my oxygen desaturation index (ODI) was below 80%.

Sleep apnoea is a severe sleep disorder that happens when your breathing stops and starts while you sleep. If untreated, it can cause loud snoring, daytime tiredness, or more severe problems like heart trouble or high blood pressure.

When oxygen levels fall below 80%, the body can release adrenaline, which triggers the following changes in the body:

- increasing the heart rate, which may lead to a feeling of the heart racing
- redirecting blood toward the muscles, causing a surge in energy or shaking limbs

- relaxing the airways to give the muscles more oxygen, which may cause breathing to become shallow

What was happening to me was that I would wake up in the morning having trashed the bed. The sheets would be wet from perspiration, and it looked like five people had been wrestling in the bed all night.

A second test with Resmed confirmed my diagnosis, and I was strongly recommended to purchase a device and use it every night.

The day I first used my new Resmed Sleep Apnoea machine, I slept like a baby and woke up in the same position I remember going to sleep. I don't think I moved all night, so restful was my sleep.

Jacqui, however, hardly slept all night and has often told how she sat alongside our bed and watched to see if I was asleep and not dead.

2014: Attempted Suicide

I had been under a lot of pressure with work and finance problems at this time, and like most men, I kept it to myself and just tried to push through the darkness threatening to engulf me.

While I thought this approach had worked for me for several years, I now believe the pressure built and built until the day I snapped, and Jacqui passed a comment that, at that time, was enough to push me over the edge. While I won't tell you how I tried to take my life, I will describe the events unfolding.

I drove around for a few hours, contemplating running my car into a tree at speed, but I could not find a suitable place without risking someone else's life. So, I purchased what I needed to get the job done and drove to a nearby reserve where I could sit in my car without being interrupted. I had a bottle of Gin, which I thought would give me the courage to do what I was planning, and it caused me to be what I would describe as melancholy.

Apparently, I started texting Jacqui to say I was sorry. The text messages were gibberish, as I was so intoxicated that I could not type coherently. The following things made it difficult, if not impossible, for Jacqui to figure out where I was.

- At no time did I give Jacqui my location.
- I was parked off the street in a car park in a different suburb to the one we lived in

- I was parked in a location we had never frequented
- The place I parked was randomly selected and deliberately out of the way
- I did not have a tracking system that would allow anyone to find me

Despite these facts, Jacqui somehow figured out where I was from my responses and called an ambulance. I remember her opening the car door and saying, "Robert, what have you done?".

Those words are as fresh in my mind today as they were then, and as the ambulance officers pulled me out of the car and placed me in the ambulance, those words got louder and louder until I passed out.

I woke up hours later in Westmead Hospital ICU with Jacqui sitting by my bed.

I was ashamed of what I had done. I was even more embarrassed that I had failed, and it soon became apparent that the doctors and nurses who knew viewed me with contempt, or at least that's how I saw it at the time.

Then came the psychologists who, before discharging me, wanted to know what I had done, why I had tried to do it, and, importantly, I would try again.

Ever the salesperson, I quickly figured out what they needed me to tell them before discharging me. So I told them what they wanted to hear, and I was allowed to go home a few days later.

What I didn't know and only found out recently was that the psychiatrist rang Jacqui and quizzed her on the condition in the house and how I would be supported if I were discharged. They were concerned about the prospects of being left unattended, how Jacqui and my daughters felt about my attempted suicide and what steps the family would take to ensure I received the help I needed.

After being discharged, I agreed to see a psychologist to placate everyone concerned. The selection of a suitable person was left up to us, so after talking with Jacqui, we decided I would see a person we both knew from our church.

As it turned out, this was a poor choice from a mental health perspective. The familiarity with this person forced me to be a little selective about what I chose to talk to him about, while from his perspective, I am sure the professional relationship was constrained.

While the sessions with this psychologist helped a little, I failed to make any real progress in dealing with my feelings and the constant depression that consumed me day and night. After several weeks of seeing this psychologist, we concluded that there was nothing further to be gained from our sessions, so we agreed to end the sessions.

I never discussed it with that psychologist, but I thought I was never alone and was constantly being watched from that point onwards. The home was never going to be the same again.

When you suffer from depression, you want to be alone; you don't want to talk about what happened, and you don't feel like going out because of the likelihood that you will run into people.

People didn't know how to approach me or what to say, so keeping a distance was the best way to handle the situation. I didn't want to discuss my breakdown more than they did, but I saw their avoidance as rejection, further fuelling my depression.

People I thought were friends kept their distance from me, and the people I love, my family, didn't know how to handle the situation. It hurt when I was on my own and out and about, and no matter what I did, I felt I was losing my mind.

Around this time, Jacqui's father passed away, and we decided to move in with Jacqui's mother, who was not coping with Peter's death. The arrangement was complicated, and at the time, I formed the opinion that we were living there so Judy could keep an eye on me rather than being there to support her.

2014: Planned Suicide

Living with my mother-in-law was not complicated because she was only eight years older, so we had similar viewpoints on many things and got on reasonably well.

I was still struggling with my depression but putting on a good front, given that I had passed the test of my first psychologist.

I decided the best way, even the coward's, was not to kill myself but walk into the bush, get seriously lost and let events unfold for me. Given the number of people lost in the bush, Katoomba was the logical choice, so I took a train trip to Katoomba.

The train timetable was easy to access on my phone, so I looked it up and figured out when I needed to leave home to get to Katoomba with enough time to walk off into the bush and be far enough into the valley before nightfall.

I left my phone, keys and wallet at home, walked to the local train station and caught the train to Central Station. From there, it was a matter of finding the platform for Katoomba, and I would be on my way.

Sitting on the train waiting to depart, I dozed off to sleep for a while and was woken by an intercom announcement saying the train was out of commission and everyone would have to change to a different train on another platform.

This delay in train departure would change the time I arrived at Katoomba, which put my plans into chaos. It would have been too late to walk as far into the bush before nightfall as I had planned, and I didn't want to have the choice of being able to hike back out of the bush. I wanted to be lost in the bush when the sun went down. So the logical thing was to return home and do this another day when the trains didn't break down.

When I arrived home, because I didn't have keys to the house and no one was home, I just climbed over the side gate and sat outside in the backyard. Thirty minutes passed, and my sister-in-law opened the back door and said, "where have you been?". Jacqui has been frantic about where you are and what you have done.

It turns out Jacqui has a friend in the police force, and between them, they decided to look at the history of my phone's internet browser to see if there were any clues. They found the train timetable in Katoomba and alerted the Katoomba Police and our local police. They tracked me via CCT footage on the local and Central Stations in the city but could not confirm whether I had boarded the Katoomba train.

The police were waiting for me at Katoomba, and when I didn't get off the train, they started backtracking to see where I may have gone.

A short time after my sister-in-law told Jacqui I was home, the police arrived and wanted to know where I had been and what I had been doing. I talked my way out of that situation and was watched closely for the next few weeks.

Soon after, I was convinced I needed to see a psychologist to get help because everyone was convinced I would try suicide again. After a heated discussion with Jacqui, I caved in and agreed to see this person she had been seeing.

2015: Diabetes

I was diagnosed with type-2 diabetes with acute high blood sugar levels, and this condition was undiagnosed for over ten years.

Type-2 diabetes is when the body becomes resistant to the usual effects of insulin and gradually loses the capacity to produce enough insulin in the pancreas. The condition has genetic and family-related risk factors and is often associated with modifiable lifestyle risk factors.

Type-2 diabetes remission as an HbA1c of under 6.5% (48mmol/mol) for at least three months without glucose-lowering medications.

Diabetes and Complications

Diabetes mellitus (DM), commonly known as just diabetes, is a group of metabolic disorders characterised by a high blood sugar level over a prolonged period.

Symptoms often include frequent urination, increased thirst, and increased appetite.

If left untreated, diabetes can cause many health complications. Acute complications can include diabetic ketoacidosis, hyperosmolar hyperglycemic state, or death.

Long-term complications include cardiovascular disease, stroke, chronic kidney disease, foot ulcers, nerve damage, eyes, and cognitive impairment.

Diabetes is due to either the pancreas not producing enough insulin or the body's cells not responding correctly to the insulin produced. There are three main types of diabetes mellitus:

- *Type-1 diabetes results from the failure of the pancreas to produce enough insulin due to the loss of beta cells. This form was previously referred to as "insulin-dependent diabetes mellitus" (IDDM) or "juvenile diabetes". An autoimmune response causes the loss of beta cells. The cause of this autoimmune response is unknown.*
- *Type-2 diabetes begins with insulin resistance, in which cells fail to respond to insulin appropriately. This form was previously referred to as "non-insulin-dependent diabetes mellitus" (NIDDM) or "adult-onset diabetes". The most common cause is a combination of excessive body weight and insufficient exercise. As the disease progresses, a lack of insulin may also develop.*
- *Gestational diabetes is the third main form and occurs when pregnant women without an earlier history of diabetes develop high blood sugar levels.*

According to Diabetes Research Clinical Practice

As of 2019, an estimated 463 million people had diabetes worldwide (8.8% of the adult population), with type-2 diabetes making up about 90% of the cases. Rates are similar in women and men. Trends suggest that rates will continue to rise.

Diabetes at least doubles a person's risk of early death. In 2019, diabetes resulted in approximately 4.2 million deaths. It is the seventh leading cause of death globally. The global economic cost of diabetes-related health expenditure in 2017 was estimated at US$727 billion. In the United States, diabetes cost nearly US$327 billion in 2017.

So, by now, you have started to get the picture right. Health in decline, family and friends look on in disbelief as my health continuously moves in the wrong direction.

2015: Peripheral Neuropathy

Ten years undiagnosed as a person with type-2 diabetes with blood sugar readings over 20 caused severe damage to the peripheral nerves in my legs and hands.

My next specialist was a neurologist who, after testing the nerves in my legs and arms, advised that I was suffering from a condition called Peripheral Neuropathy and as if the news couldn't get any better, she told me I would experience acute nerve pain requiring strong medication to cope with the pain. You could imagine the joy of being told I would see my leg muscles slowly shrink away and how to drop foot would be the next stage of the illness before ultimately losing the use of my legs and being a wheelchair user for the rest of my life.

Your peripheral nervous system connects the nerves from your brain and spinal cord, or central nervous system, to the rest of your body. In my case, the nerves in my legs were not working correctly, sending signals of pain when nothing was causing pain and not sending pain signals when something was causing harm.

I first noticed changes in my legs with a simple nerve twitch. The frequency of twitching increased, and I started to feel a sensation I can only describe as being stabbed with an ice pick.

Next came the feeling of numbness from my hips down while standing. Walking helped improve the condition for some time, but eventually, that feeling of numbness grew more consistent.

Finally, when I cut my foot outside in the backyard, Jacqui told me I was bleeding as I walked into the house. Jacqui looked at the cut and found a burr the size of a small button wedged between two of my toes. I looked around; on the white tiles in our family room, I could see this blood trail from the back door.

My toes were infected, and only after removing the burr was the severity of the damage to my foot evident.

From my perspective, I struggled to keep my balance in the dark. With a lack of feeling in my feet and numbness in my legs, my balance was compromised when I could not use my eyes to help maintain my balance. I struggled to stand in a pitch-black room without losing balance and would reach out for anything that helped me maintain balance.

The doctor prescribed a beautiful little drug called Lyrica, initially developed for treating epilepsy and acts as a central nerve blocker. Given the intense pain, the fantastic drug eased the pain considerably.

Lyrica has since been described as addictive and, over time, requires a higher dose to continue effectively suppressing the pain.

For several years, I struggled with the pain, and while Lyrica was a wonder drug, it was not until I decided to come off the medicine that I realised how addictive it was.

I experienced withdrawal symptoms that manifested as rage and anger, and I had difficulty controlling my temper only after two days without taking the drug. After retaking the medication, I noticed the pain had reduced, but I remained angry and quick to temper for almost a week.

Finally, because of Lyrica, I believe my cognitive capabilities were reduced. Sometimes, the most straightforward problems seemed to be an issue for me, so I wondered if I was also suffering from Alzheimer's.

In April 2023, I finally stopped taking Lyrica and slowly reduced the medication by halving it every two weeks for several months.

Overview of Peripheral Neuropathy

Peripheral neuropathy is caused by damage to the nerves outside the brain and spinal cord (peripheral nerves), often causing weakness, numbness and pain, usually in the hands and feet. It can also affect other areas and body functions, including digestion, urination, and circulation.

Your peripheral nervous system sends information from your brain and spinal cord (central nervous system) to the rest of your body. The peripheral nerves also send sensory information to the central nervous system.

Peripheral neuropathy can result from many different illnesses, but it was caused by diabetes, in my instance.

I experience stabbing, burning and tingling pain lasting several hours. The medication that has proved most effective in reducing my pain has been Lyrica.

Symptoms

Every nerve in your peripheral system has a specific function, so symptoms depend on the type of nerves affected. Nerves are classified into:

- Sensory nerves that receive sensation, such as temperature, pain, vibration or touch, from the skin
- Motor nerves that control muscle movement
- Autonomic nerves that control functions such as blood pressure, perspiration, heart rate, digestion and bladder function

Signs and symptoms of peripheral neuropathy might include:
- Loss of balance
- Lack of coordination and falling
- Numbness, prickling or tingling in your feet or hands
- Sharp, jabbing, throbbing or burning pain
- Extreme sensitivity to touch
- Muscle weakness
- Feeling as if you're wearing gloves or socks when you're not
- Paralysis if motor nerves are affected

2018: Stroke

Flash forward to 2018, and after an average night's sleep standing in front of the bathroom mirror first thing in the morning, the left side of my face had fallen, and when I touched my cheek and lips, they were numb. It was clear the stroke had affected my thinking because instead of calling for an ambulance or going to the hospital, I decided to call my family doctor, so I called to make an appointment.

The young woman on the other end of the phone advised that the practice was not open yet and asked if I could call back. I explained that I thought I had had a stroke, and she responded, "hang on a moment; I will get a doctor for you".

The doctor advised me to come to the surgery immediately, so I hung up the phone and told Jacqui we needed to go to the doctor's surgery.

When we arrived, the surgery was shut, so we knocked on the door. Someone came to the door and advised us that the surgery would not be open for twenty minutes. When I explained that I had called earlier and had been told to come in immediately, we were told they had had no calls and provided no such advice. I was so, off my game due to the stroke; the doctor I called was not my regular doctor but a different doctor's surgery I had never visited before.

Standing twenty metres away, my doctor could see and hear what was happening, so she ushered us into the surgery. After a quick check, she told me we had two choices: drive to Norwest Emergency, or she could call an ambulance.

We decided to drive to Northwest Hospital as it was a five-minute drive, but we changed our mind and headed to Westmead Hospital because Jacqui believed they were better equipped to handle the situation.

The stroke was confirmed later that day, and I called it my Lucky Stroke because it turned out to be a mild stroke, and I fully recovered.

After a week in Westmead Hospital, several tests, lots of therapy and a medication change, I could go home. My lucky stroke gave me the wake-up call to start caring more for myself and my health than I had been doing.

The decision to get medical help was right, but my choice of who should have been was inconsistent with the current recommendation for stroke sufferers. CALL AN AMBULANCE.

What is a Stroke

A stroke occurs when your brain can't get enough oxygen and essential nutrients, usually because a blood clot or sudden bleed reduces the blood supply.

What are the signs of a stroke? If you or someone you are with shows signs of having a stroke pay particular attention and note when the symptoms began. Some treatment options are most effective when given soon after a stroke starts.

Signs and symptoms of stroke include:

- *Trouble speaking and understanding what others are saying. You may experience confusion, slur your words or have difficulty understanding speech.*
- *Paralysis or numbness of the face, arm or leg. You may develop sudden numbness, weakness, or paralysis in your face, arm, or leg, often affecting just one side of your body. Try to raise both your arms over your head at the same time. If one arm begins to fall, you may be having a stroke. Also, one side of your mouth may droop when you try to smile.*
- *Problems are seen in one or both eyes. You may suddenly have blurred or blackened vision in one or both eyes or see double.*
- *Headache. A sudden, severe headache, accompanied by vomiting, dizziness or altered consciousness, may indicate that you're having a stroke.*
- *Trouble walking. You may stumble or lose your balance. You may also have sudden dizziness or a loss of coordination.*

***Call 000** or your local emergency number right away. Don't wait to see if symptoms stop. Every minute counts. The longer a stroke goes untreated, the greater the potential for brain damage and disability.*

If you're with someone you suspect has a stroke, observe the person while waiting for emergency assistance.

2019: Collapse Lung Pneumonia

In December 2019, Jacqui and I went on our first cruise together and enjoyed cruising the south pacific.

Within days of getting off the ship, I suffered from what we believed was a severe cold/flu bug, except I could not shake it.

My doctor decided she needed X-rays, so a quick trip down the road and back to the doctor revealed I had a collapsed lung and pneumonia.

There were no real complications, just two weeks of rest and some potent antibiotics, but it all cleared up, and there have been no more issues since.

2021: Enlarged Prostate

After one of my regular blood screening tests showed a larger-than-expected increase in my PSA (prostate-specific antigen) Reading, my doctor sent me to a urologist.

After discussing the number of times I had to get out of bed in the night to urinate (three to four times a night), my urologist performed my first rectal examination. There were no noticeable irregularities, but the frequency of my urination and the reduced flow caused the need for another medication to help improve the flow.

After having an ultrasound on my prostate, it was determined that I had one of the biggest prostates in the southern hemisphere.

My urologist suggested having my waterworks bored out (pipes cleaned and enlarged). After a bit of thought, I decided to live with the inconvenience.

Given that I was trying to reduce the number of medications I was taking daily, I decided not to have the prescription filled but to cope as best I could with the need to urinate more frequently than the average man.

The PSA test is the leading method of screening for prostate cancer. PSA screening can help catch the disease early when treatment may be more effective and potentially have fewer side effects. The PSA test may be done with a digital rectal exam, in which a physician inserts a gloved finger into the rectum to examine the prostate for irregularities.

What Does PSA Stand For?

PSA, or prostate-specific antigen, is a protein produced by the prostate and mainly found in semen, with tiny amounts released into the bloodstream. More PSA is released when there's a problem with the prostate—such as the development and growth of prostate cancer.

But you can say "no more" to symptoms like waking up at night to urinate and having the urgent need to go. Or a weak stream. Left untreated, it can lead to more serious urinary, bladder and kidney problems.

The actual cause of prostate enlargement is unknown. Factors linked to ageing and changes in the cells of the testicles may have a role in the growth of the gland and testosterone levels. Men who have had their testicles removed at a young age due to testicular cancer do not develop enlarged prostates.

Some Facts About Prostate Enlargement

- *The likelihood of developing an enlarged prostate increases with age.*
- *BPH is so common that it has been said that all men will have an enlarged prostate if they live long enough.*

- *A small amount of prostate enlargement exists in many men over age forty. More than 90% of men over age eighty have the condition.*
- *No risk factors have been identified other than having normally functioning testicles.*

2021: Cardiovascular Disease

The struggle most of us have with the concept of chest pain is because we are never really sure when that pain is significant enough to warrant seeing a doctor or, worse still, calling an ambulance.

From my perspective, I would have called it more discomfort than pain, but when you add other factors into the equation, like feeling light-headed and whiteout when you stand up, you need to bite the bullet and see your doctor.

My doctor instantly pushed me into the nurse's room and had an ECG performed.

The ECG was inconclusive, but again, my doctor operated on the side of caution every time and rang the cardiologist she usually recommends. She told them she had a patient in her room, and wanted the cardiologist to see them with some urgency.

Ten minutes later, I was sitting in his waiting room, and within thirty minutes, I was sitting in front of that doctor.

Five minutes later, I walked on their stress machine and connected to another ECG device as the incline gradually increased, pushing harder and harder to the point I could go no higher.

An appointment with an imaging service, radioactive dye and a full MRI scan of my heart later, the cardiologist advised that I had cardiovascular disease and needed to be admitted to the hospital for a day surgery angiogram.

The scan report showed a Coronary Artery Calcium Score of 725.9, indicating the presence of a severe identifiable plaque burden. Generally, a score >50 is problematic, but a score >400 means you have a plaque build-up, and your risk of a heart attack in the next five years is high.

One week later, I was admitted to Norwest Private Hospital for an angiogram, which showed my arteries had a 40% blockage; as such, I did not require stents or bypass surgery; however, my medication was changed to include the use of a Statin to reduce the risk of heart attack and stroke and Clopidogrel, a platelet inhibitor to reduce the chance of blood clots.

2022: Kidney Disease

As part of my research for this book, I obtained all of my blood test reports dating back to 2000. As a result of this research, I have been suffering from kidney disease, fluctuating between stage 1 and stage 3b, the realisation that my last test results showed stage 3b with an increased probability of kidney failure and a short life expectancy. The conclusion was that my life expectancy would be reduced, and the likelihood of needing regular dialysis was unacceptable unless I could reverse this condition.

I was not looking forward to my doctor's appointment that day. The kidney functionality test results from my blood test that week would either confirm an improvement or the realisation that life was about to take a downward trend.

While the human body has a remarkable capacity to repair itself, all the research I have done up until today indicated it was impossible. For that reason, I was filled with doubt and anxiety.

As you will see in the blood test results highlighted in the next section, the result was an outstanding improvement.

Not only have I been able to reverse the downward spiral of my kidney health, but my weight loss and health improvement activities have elevated the threshold associated with kidney disease. My kidneys have repaired themselves and are functioning correctly for the first time in twenty years.

2022: Prostate Cancer

After one of my regular blood tests two years ago, my doctor pointed out that my PSA results showed another out-of-character increase compared to my previous test results. Hence, she referred me back to my urologist.

The test showed a dramatic increase in my PSA levels. While the results were still in range for my age, the significant change was four times greater than average for twelve months, which warranted further examination.

After the polite conversation, excluding dinner and a glass of excellent wine, we went straight to digital penetration. After examining my prostate using this much-revered technique, my urologist advised that he could feel an abnormality that warranted further examination, so he scheduled an MRI to confirm his suspicions.

PSA (Prostate-Specific Antigen) is a protein made in the prostate gland. The prostate is a walnut-sized gland below the bladder in front of the rectum. It surrounds the urethra, the passage in the penis through which urine and semen pass.

PSA is produced by prostate cells and enters the bloodstream. As men age and the prostate gland grows more prominent, they can often make higher levels of PSA. However, higher levels of PSA can also be caused by other conditions. One of these is prostate cancer.

I went back to my urologist to get the results of my MRI; I found myself sitting there expecting the results would not be great, so I spent the first few minutes talking to him about his holidays to the Whitsundays. While I was not overly interested in his holiday, it helped me build a relationship while preparing my head for what I felt would be bad news.

The report shows the MRI found three lesions, "PI-RADS 5 ", which is the highest reading and indicates the most severe probability of cancer. He told me that "5 is very suspicious"; based on that result, we need to perform a biopsy on the lesions.

My urologist scheduled two procedures for day surgery: a biopsy of the three lesions and a Rigid Cystoscopy.

A prostate biopsy is a procedure to remove samples of suspicious tissue from the prostate using a needle to collect tissue samples from your prostate gland.

The rigid cystoscopy is a procedure used to check for any problems in your bladder using a rigid telescope inserted into the penis via the urethra and into the bladder. This process allows the urologist to fix issues with your bladder and the urinary tubes connecting the kidneys to the bladder.

One week later, with Jacqui to support me, we returned to get the biopsy results.

Preparing myself for this meeting was simple; I just imagined the worst possible scenario and researched the internet to determine what would be required surgically.

I was advised that I would have blood in my urine for a week after the procedure; the amount of blood and the fact that it continued bleeding for twelve days led me to conclude that the urologist had taken a biopsy from my bladder and prostate.

If the assumption that I had bladder and prostate cancer were correct, it would require the removal of my bladder, a bowel resection to use part of the bowel to act as an alternative bladder and the permanent use of a colostomy tube and urine bag.

After the surgery, I would require several chemotherapy treatments to remove any other metastasised growth that may have set up camp in my body. So, as you can imagine, anything less would be a bonus.

I believed that preparing myself for the worst possible news of having bladder and prostate cancer was my way of dealing with the inevitable bad news. My rationalisation for this belief was based on the idea that anything less than bladder and prostate cancer was something that I could cope with and get my life back on track.

The consultation started well with the usual idle chit-chat before getting down to the nitty-gritty.

From a prostate cancer perspective, they use a grade from 1-4 to categorise the severity of cancer.

'Robert, unfortunately, we have found you have several cancers, which have been graded as 1, 2, 3 and 4, while the one we graded as 4 has already spread beyond the prostate.'

My doctor advised that he wanted me to have a PET Scan performed to identify any metastases that have already started to grow in other parts of my body. You will need to have the prostate removed, and we will need to remove your lymph glands simultaneously.

Cancer is a word we hear frequently and don't think we will ever hear as part of a medical prognosis delivered to us by a doctor. Having lost my mother and stepfather to lung cancer and watching Mum go through two rounds of chemotherapy was an experience that will live in my memory forever.

The PET scan uses a special dye containing radioactive tracers injected into a vein in your arm, depending on what part of the body is examined. Specific organs and tissues then absorb the tracer.

When detected by a PET scanner, the tracers help your doctor see how well your organs and tissues work. In contrast, the tracer collects in areas of higher chemical activity, which is helpful because specific tissues of the body and certain diseases have a higher level of chemical activity. These disease areas show up as bright spots on the PET scan.

After ten days of grappling with negative thoughts and trying my hardest to stay positive, Jacqui and I finally met with the urologist, who advised that the PET scan had found no other metaseries outside the fatty tissue surrounding the prostate. From this point onwards, all we needed to do was set a surgery date and prepare me for the operation.

Preparations for prostate surgery are simple: a referral to a physiotherapist and some exercises to strengthen my pelvic floor.

Wrong!

Multiple visits to the physio and fourteen different exercises to help strengthen the three muscles we use to stop the urine flow before you shake those lost few droplets from the end of your penis. Three muscles, really; why could we not just have one muscle to do that? Then, the exercises could have been cut by two-thirds.

The physio holds an ultrasound device between your testicles and anus while he tells you to use the muscles as the expression goes, "Lift your cock". Then you see these three muscles working with the aid of ultrasound while standing there with your shorts around your knees. The three muscles contract in three directions to strangle your urethra and stop the urine flow, an experience I hope most of you never have to endure.

Radical prostatectomy includes removing the entire prostate gland, capsule, surrounding lymph nodes and neighbouring tissue and can be performed using one of three different surgical procedures.

Open Prostatectomy

The surgeon accesses the prostate gland through a standard surgical incision in the open surgical procedure. For most patients, the incision is ten to twelve centimetres long.

Laparoscopic Radical Prostatectomy

The surgeon inserts special long instruments through several small incisions in the abdominal wall to remove the prostate.

Robotic Prostatectomy

This operation is performed under general anaesthetic. The three-dimensional robotic camera and robotic arms are inserted through small (eight mm) incisions in the abdomen. The surgeon controls the arms via a remote console in the operating theatre. The prostate is dissected free from the bladder and surrounding structures. The bladder is then joined to the urethra over a catheter tube. This catheter will remain in place for seven days while the reconnection of the urethra heals.

9 July 2022, Three Days Before Surgery

Jacqui and I had tickets to a two-and-a-half-day conference in Newcastle, which we had purchased before I was diagnosed with prostate cancer. Given the difficulties with COVID-19, we decided I would not attend the conference as I needed to isolate myself before being hospitalised. To support Jacqui, we decided to travel to Newcastle together. I would spend the time Jacqui was in the conference sessions getting some fresh air and exercise while dealing with my negative thoughts about the upcoming surgery.

On Saturday, I had an unusual experience believing that I needed to urinate, except all I passed was about 100 mils of old blood. After the biopsy, I had been advised that I would see some bleeding and that this would stop after a few weeks, but given several weeks had passed since that procedure, I was a little freaked out. On top of this, a friend texted me to be supportive while letting me know he would pray for me. The text message advised that I should take Jacqui out for a nice romantic dinner because, after my surgery, *I would not be able to satisfy my wife sexually again.*

With the best of intentions, I have no doubt, but telling me something I already knew and when I was trying hard to push all the negative thoughts out of my head was not what I needed.

The loss of blood followed by the text message took me down the proverbial rabbit hole that the blood loss was a sign of a bigger problem—at the same time, confirming that my masculinity, my ability ever to satisfy a woman in the usual way, would be cut out of my body.

My urologist had told me that the removal of the prostate gland would result in my inability to ejaculate, given the ejaculation fluid is manufactured in the prostate. He also advised that the nerves associated with arousal and the sensations in the penis that lead to ejaculation would most likely be damaged and that I would never experience the sexual arousal and gratification I was accustomed to experiencing.

In short, given I had already had a vasectomy, urination would be the only function of my penis after the surgery was a massive issue for me as a man, as I believe it would be for all men. To make matters worse, the ability to urinate, or should I say, control my urination, was going to be compromised.

Pelvic Floor Physiotherapy Training

My urologist referred me to a physiotherapist who provided pelvic floor training exercises to assist with the ability to control urination post-surgery. To understand the significance of the need to do these exercises, one must appreciate the anatomical differences between pre-surgery and post-surgery.

The prostate is a male reproductive system gland between the bladder and penis.

The urethra is a tube connected to the bladder and the penis, which allows us to pass urine.

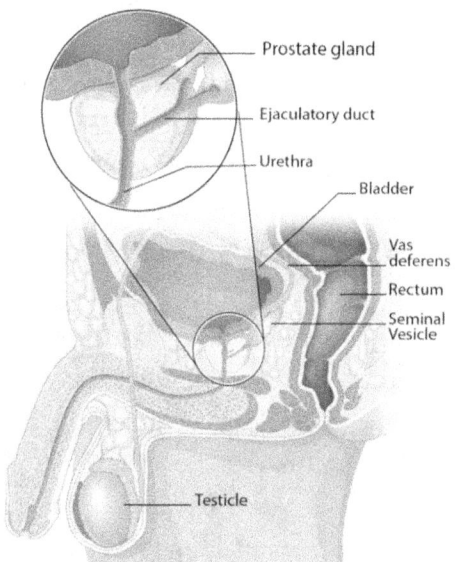

During a radical prostatectomy, a surgeon removes the entire prostate gland and a section of the urethra that passes through the prostate. The remaining section of the urethra is then reconnected to the bladder. A catheter is then inserted to allow urine to drain from the bladder for seven days while the urethra connection to the bladder heals.

Pelvic floor exercises improve a person's ability to control incontinence after surgery. When enlarged prostates, seminal vesicles, and lymph nodes are removed, gravity and vacated space allow the bladder to return to its original size and capacity. These factors, combined with damaged nerves and weakened pelvic floor muscles, contribute to the need to urinate urgently and for what is best described as bladder leakage.

The inability to control urination was significantly reduced, and the need to wear male nappies and incontinence pads was always going to be a hurdle for me and an inspiration to do whatever was required to retrain my body and gain control of my bodily functions. The exercises were straightforward, but following the instruction provided by my physiotherapist allowed me to, as he put it, advance myself well and truly beyond the curve.

Recovery from prostate cancer surgery has its difficulties, but the greatest one for me was the requirement to walk no more than twelve minutes, building to fifteen minutes a day for the first four weeks. It was complicated because I had become accustomed to rising at 5:00 am seven days a week and walking ten to fourteen kilometres before breakfast. Anatomically, the reason for restricting the amount of walking, standing and sitting is straightforward. With a significantly enlarged prostate removed, the bladder loses its cushion, which a void replaces. Combined with a shorter urethra pulling on a surgically attached connection to the bladder, it needs time to heal and adjust to the void.

Sitting and lying down for weeks and extending into months was always going to be an issue for me, so I pushed the limits of what I was required to do compared to what I was accustomed to doing as part of my daily habits.

Finally, coming to grips with the realisation that my ability to gain a full erection and never experience the sexual gratification that I have become accustomed to is a hurdle I will navigate over the rest of my life. While I no longer have a seminal vesicle or vas deferens that connect to my urethral that manufacture and mix sperm and seminal fluid that make ejaculate, the ability to experience ejaculation has now been removed from my sex life.

I am struggling with this new reality, given I am no longer a man as God made me but rather a eunuch.

Understanding Blood Test Results

Date	2/01/2000	28/09/2009	31/10/2018	22/10/2019	11/12/2019	10/07/2020	24/11/2020	3/09/2021	10/03/2022	29/04/2022	27/07/2022	7/08/2023	21/02/2024	8/04/2024	Units	Range
Time F-Fast	Unkn F	Unkn F	Unkn F					Unkn F	Unkn F		Fast	Fast		Fast		
Lab ID	95253106	49288854	841685548	841685548	841685548	49288854	49288854	49288854	49288854	880864872	969390497	884963938	836284821	836284821		
Status	Fasting	Fasting						Fasting	Fasting					Fasting		
Sodium	140	140	146	142	144	144	141	142		145	143	144	143	142	mmol/L	(135-145)
Potassium	3.9	4.5	4.8	4.9	3.9	4.5	4.2	4.2		3.9	3.9	4.9	4.2	3.9	mmol/L	(3.5-5.5)
Chloride	105	106	108	105	109	107	110	107		108	105	108	105	104	mmol/L	(98-110)
Bicarbonate	25	27	23	28	26	31	24	27		25	24	27	30	28	mmol/L	(20-32)
Urea	8.4	7.0	12	10.2	8.1	6.3	7.1	9.3		7.1	8.3	8.9	7.6	8.7	mmol/L	(3.5-9.0)
Creatinine	125	140	150	150	135	115	120	130		95	115	100	115	100	umol/L	(60-110)
eGFR	61	44	39	40	45	55	52	46	60	67	53	62	55	62	mL/min	(>59)
Uric Acid		0.34				0.32		0.36		15				0.26	mmol/L	(0.20-0.50)
Calcium	2.40	2.43						2.51		74					mmol/L	(2.15-2.55)
Corr Calcium	2.28	2.39								14					mmol/L	(2.15-2.55)
Phosphate	1.14	0.93						1.06		251					mmol/L	(0.8-1.5)
Bili.Total	16	14	16	24	18	26	18	34		19	15	25	19	22	umol/L	(4-20)
ALP	76	73	107	98	109	93	87	75		74	65	71	69		U/L	(35-110)
GGT	39	27	20	15	25	13	13	13		14	9	13	14		U/L	(5-50)
LDH	249	243	212	329	250	214	214	323		256	351	379	271	293	U/L	(120-250)
AST	52	39	35	32	37	36	32	44		61	48	51	53	58	U/L	(10-40)
ALT	58	38	33	25	35	29	25	31		36	36	37	48	49	U/L	(5-40)
Total Protein	77	76	74	71	76	74	71	72		71	72	67	72	72	g/L	(64-83)
Albumin	46	45	43	43	43	45	43	48		46	44	44	45	48	g/L	(36-47)
Globulin	31	31	31	28	33	29	28	24		25	28	23	27	24	g/L	(23-39)
Cholesterol	4.1	4.3				2.8		2.9		3		3.3		3.5	mmol/L	(3.9-6.5)
Triglycerides	1.8	1.5				2		0.6		1.8		0.5		0.6	mmol/L	(0.5-1.7)
CK								390		279	547	365	316	358	U/L	(40-200)
PSA	0.8	1.1					2.2	2.6	4.4	0.01	0.01	0.01		0.01		Age 40-49: 0-2.5 ng/m; 50-59: 0-3.5 ng/m; 60-69: 0-4.5 ng/m; 70-79: 0-6.5 ng/m
Insulin																
Fasting		7.3														(3.6-6.0)
1 Hour		13.5														(3.6-6.0)
2 Hours		11.3														(3.6-7.7)
HbA1c			22.1	12.2	9.8	8.8	5.9	4.8	5.6			5.8	5.8	5.5		(3.8-6.0)
Weight	139.7kg	137.6kg		138.6kg	138.2kg	137.9kg	118.7kg	104.2kg			99.7		100.2			

In the summary table of my blood tests, as shown above, the extent of my kidney disease was at an all-time low in 2019, showed some improvement by 2019 and fell away by November 2020 before crashing again in September 2021 to an all-time high low and Stage 3b kidney disease.

The eFGR results are consistently lower than (>59), indicating my kidney function has entered Stage 3b of the five stages of kidney disease. The point of end-stage renal disease and death are the likely conclusions.

Sodium

Sodium is an electrolyte essential in regulating water levels and other bodily substances. When sodium levels in the blood become too low, it leads to hyponatraemia, causing lethargy, confusion, and fatigue.

Potassium

A potassium test may be recommended to help diagnose or monitor kidney disease, the most common cause of high potassium levels. Your doctor may also recommend the test if you have heart-related problems, such as high blood pressure (hypertension).

Chloride

Chloride is one of the electrolytes in your blood. Many factors can cause an abnormal chloride level in your blood, including dehydration, vomiting and certain medical conditions. Chloride blood tests ensure you have appropriate chloride levels in your blood to be healthy.

Bicarbonate

The bicarbonate (or total CO_2) test is usually ordered along with sodium, potassium, and chloride as part of an electrolyte panel, which is included in a basic metabolic panel (BMP) and a comprehensive metabolic panel (CMP). A calculated bicarbonate level might also be reported as part of a blood gas panel.

Urea

High urea levels suggest poor kidney function. This may be due to acute or chronic kidney disease.

Creatinine

An elevated creatinine level signifies impaired kidney function or kidney disease. As the kidneys become incapacitated, the creatinine level in the blood will rise due to poor clearance of creatinine by the kidneys. Abnormally high creatinine levels thus warn of possible malfunction or failure of the kidneys.

eFGR

Stage 3 defines the point at which mortality becomes a greater concern than the likelihood of developing end-stage renal disease. With kidney function reduced between 59-30mL/min, the previously minor symptoms of stage 2 become far more severe. From the end of stage 3, only 15 points of kidney function stand between entering stage 5, which indicates total kidney failure.

Uric Acid

High uric acid levels can cause gout, and you'll need to try to lower it. If you have gout symptoms, you need to take a uric acid blood test, which measures how much uric acid you have in your blood.

Calcium

Calcium in urine test measures the amount of calcium in your urine (pee). If your urine calcium levels are too high or too low, it may be a sign of kidney disease, kidney stones, bone disease, parathyroid gland disorder, or other conditions.

Corr Calcium

A calcium blood test measures the amount of calcium in your blood. Suppose there is too much or too little calcium in the blood. In that case, it may signify various medical conditions, such as bone disease, thyroid disease, parathyroid disorders, kidney disease, and other conditions.

Phosphate

A high phosphate level is often a sign of kidney damage. It's more common in people with chronic kidney disease (CKD), especially those with end-stage kidney disease.

Bilirubin

Elevated levels may indicate liver damage or disease. Higher direct bilirubin levels in your blood may indicate your liver isn't clearing bilirubin properly. Elevated levels of indirect bilirubin may indicate other problems.

ALP

Higher-than-normal levels of ALP in your blood may indicate a health concern with your liver or gallbladder, including a blockage in your bile ducts, gallstones, cirrhosis, liver cancer, and some forms of hepatitis.

GGT

This test is used to detect diseases of the liver or bile ducts. It is also done with other tests (such as the ALT, AST, ALP, and bilirubin) to differentiate between liver or bile duct disorders and bone disease. It may also be done to screen for or monitor alcohol use.

LDH

High levels of LDH indicate some form of tissue damage. Extremely high levels of LDH could indicate severe disease or multiple organ failure. High levels of more than one isoenzyme may indicate more than one cause of tissue damage. For example, a patient with pneumonia could also have a heart attack.

AST

If your results are abnormal, it doesn't necessarily mean you have a medical condition needing treatment. High levels of AST in the blood may indicate hepatitis, cirrhosis, mononucleosis, or other liver diseases. Elevated AST levels can also indicate heart problems or pancreatitis.

ALT

ALT is most commonly increased in response to liver disease or liver damage caused by alcohol, drugs, supplements, or toxins. Other causes of high ALT include obesity, anorexia, biliary disease, muscle damage and disease, heart attack, hypothyroidism, and infections and conditions that can impair liver function.

Total Protein

Proteins are essential for the health and growth of the body's cells and tissues. A total protein test measures the amount of protein in your blood and can help diagnose several health conditions, including kidney disease.

Albumin

Albuminuria is a sign of kidney disease and means you have too much albumin in your urine. Albumin is a protein found in the blood. A healthy kidney doesn't let albumin pass from the blood into the urine. A damaged kidney allows some albumin to pass into the urine.

Globulin

The levels of specific globulins provide information about how well your immune system works. So, this test can diagnose immune system disorders, a type of cancer called multiple myeloma, and various other conditions.

Cholesterol

A complete cholesterol test is done to determine whether your cholesterol is high and to estimate your risk of heart attacks and other forms of heart disease and diseases of the blood vessels. A complete cholesterol test includes calculating four types of fats in your blood.

Triglycerides

A triglycerides test is a blood test that measures the amount of fat in your blood called triglycerides. Your body uses triglycerides for energy. High triglycerides may increase your risk of a heart attack or stroke. A triglycerides test can help you decide whether to take action to lower your risk.

CK

Levels of CK can rise after a heart attack, skeletal muscle injury, or strenuous exercise. They can also go up after drinking too much alcohol or taking certain medicines or supplements. CK is made up of 3 enzyme forms. These are CK-MB, CK-MM, and CK-BB.

PSA

The PSA test is primarily used to screen for prostate cancer. The test measures the amount of prostate-specific antigen (PSA) in your blood. PSA is a protein produced by cancerous and non-cancerous tissue in the prostate, a small gland that sits below the bladder in males.

Insulin

The insulin blood test is often used to discover the cause of hypoglycaemia (low blood sugar) and diagnose or monitor insulin resistance. Monitor the condition of people with type-2 diabetes.

Fasting: One Hour, Two Hours

A glucose tolerance test measures how well your body can absorb glucose or sugar after ingesting a given amount. Doctors use a glucose tolerance test to diagnose the various types of diabetes, particularly gestational or type-2 diabetes.

HbA1c

The haemoglobin A1c (HbA1c) test measures the blood sugar (glucose) attached to your haemoglobin. Haemoglobin is part of your red blood cells that carries oxygen from your lungs to the rest of your body. It is an important blood test indicating how well your diabetes is controlled.

The Importance of Blood Tests in Your Perspective

If you are anything like me, you sit with your doctor while they talk through the critical issues identified in your test, but don't walk away with a copy of the pathology test results.

Now, you may argue you don't need a copy of the results because if your doctor finds something, they will raise the issues with you. While this is true, I will take you back to my test results sheet and point out some simple facts.

From 2000 to 2021, my Creatinine and eGFR results showed my kidneys were in decline and bottomed out at a point where the measurement is considered a stage 3b kidney disease and heading to a point where dialysis would have been required. Importantly, dialysis is not a solution when a person's kidneys fail. It simply becomes a staging ground in preparation for kidney replacement.

When your kidney fails, your hands or feet may swell. You will feel tired and weak because your body needs clean blood to function correctly. Untreated uraemia may lead to seizures or coma and ultimately result in death. You must undergo dialysis or a kidney transplant if your kidneys stop working. People with kidney failure may survive days to weeks without dialysis, depending on their kidney function, symptoms, and overall medical condition.

Over those twenty-one years, I had several doctors at the same medical practice. It was not until I asked for a copy of all the test results and compiled them into one spreadsheet that the obvious issue became apparent.

My final comment about blood test results is, "Ignorance is not bliss; it's an abdication of your responsibility to look after your health and a lack of responsibility to your family, the people you love and those that love and care about; you".

70

Summary

While piecing together this medical history, I have had plenty of time to reflect on what happened and perhaps even why it happened to my health. Importantly, it has become apparent that the health issues I have lived through can be traced back to two simple facts.

I lived a life filled with indulgencies, and secondly, I gave no thought to the short- or long-term consequences of these indulgencies.

The research I have done into the impact of being overweight on a person's health has brought me to the conclusion that, without exception, all the illnesses I have had, except for leptospirosis, can be traced back to being overweight. Unquestionably, the compound effect of the various medical conditions increased the possibility of developing cancer, contributed to my depression and brought me to the point of trying to take my own life.

While I carried more weight than I should have, I never thought about the domino effect of the continuing decline in my health or how this would impact the quality of my life and the people I cared about and loved.

Importantly, I am not trying to build a case for the need for people to start a diet or to lose weight but to help people understand that our choices have consequences, and those consequences will impact not just you but your family and the people we love. It is about assisting people in understanding that choices matter, what we do, what we say, and that we need to be the best we can be so others don't fall into the trap; over 60% of the world population has made.

I have reclaimed my health, reduced my weight, and reversed the medical conditions that have plagued my life for the last thirty years and have been rewarded. I am healthier, fitter, and enjoying life more than I ever thought was possible. Of greater significance is that I did this at seventy-five years of age and against all the odds, and I believe if I could do this, so can anyone who is prepared just to put in the time and effort.

"Time and health are two precious assets that we don't recognise and appreciate until they have been depleted."

– Denis Waitley

Chapter 2
Life is a Gift

Anyone who followed cricket on 4 March 2022 will be remembered as the day Shane Warne, Australia's best spin bowler, died of a heart attack at fifty-two. That same week, we also lost Rod Marsh, who suffered a major heart attack a week earlier and passed away the morning of the same day.

For those who remember these two events, we went to sleep on the evening of 4 March, losing one of our greatest test keepers and waking the following day to the news of Shane Warne's death.

Both men played decisive roles in Australian Cricket, setting a standard for bowling and catching that will forever be recognised as the absolute standard of excellence.

Neither of these two great Australian sportsmen would have ever wanted to become a heart attack statistic.

From my perspective, I grew up believing that a world-class, top-level sportsperson had a much better chance of living a longer, healthier life than I would. Yet here I am, having suffered almost all of the modalities associated with obesity except for death, looking at both men and asking myself why I am still here, and they have gone.

Life is a gift, and like all gifts, sometimes they are unappreciated, misused, surrendered, taken for granted, or taken away from us.

My legacy is generational in that I want my grandchildren and great-grandchildren to appreciate the gift of LIFE, take care of it, and make sure they draw every last drop of goodness from it before it is lost forever or taken from them.

Never give up; never stop fighting for your health; your life will influence others.

I sat with a gentleman I met at a BNI meeting recently. We were both the same age, seventy-four at the time, and he stood to introduce himself after I had affirmed my reason for being in this group. This gentleman introduced himself, saying, "My name is John (name changed), and I am the before version of Robert". He was shorter than me and carried more excess weight than before I started my health journey, and it was clear that he had health issues.

After the meeting, we had a coffee and talked about his health. Three generations lived in one house, and all had health issues caused by being overweight. John lived with a daughter who had recently had gastric banding to help her lose weight, while her son was overweight and had type-1 diabetes.

As we talked a little more, John told me he was suffering from depression and potentially self-harming by his admission. I told him I understood how he felt and explained that I had walked in his shoes and attempted suicide once and planned a second attempt before finding someone to help me navigate the rough patch.

Three generations of excess weight have a high probability of being extended to a fourth generation if John's grandson had children.

Apart from being overweight and clinically depressed, John had arthritis, gout, high blood pressure, and kidney issues and was likely to become another heart attack statistic. But what impacted me more than anything else was that John didn't believe he could reverse his medical conditions; he didn't think he could lead a healthier life. He didn't consider that the potential improvement in his health could impact his family's generational health.

We are examples to others, good, bad or indifferent, but still examples, and as such, we can make a difference, but it has to start with us!

None of us had a say in the gift of life given to us by our parents. We were conceived in a moment of passion, imprisoned for nine months, and finally ejected into this world from the comfort of our mother's womb.

DNA from our parents created our life, yet my wife, Jacqui, reminded me during our morning walk together. I am a one-in-a-million creation because if any other egg or sperm had collided, I would have been a different person or born in a different time zone.

Jacqui and I have three daughters, and yes, I was at one stage prepared to consider trying for a fourth in the hope of having a son. Jacqui reminded me that three daughters were, because of my contribution, sperm with the X chromosome. I was not happy with her explanation. I did my research, which I have included below for interested people.

As for what determines our sex, women have a genetic combination of XX, and men have XY. Women provide each egg with an X. Each sperm can be an X or a Y. If the fertilised egg and sperm combine an X and Y, it's a boy. If there are two Xs, it's a girl.

The human DNA is organised into shapes you may have seen in drawings and photos called chromosomes. They resemble a wobbly letter X. Each person has forty-six, twenty-three from each parent. One pair is the sex chromosomes, known as the X and Y, and as discussed previously, they determine the baby's sex.

Of the twenty-three pairs, twenty-two are known as autosomes. The twenty-third pair comprises the sex "X" and "Y" chromosomes. This pair of chromosomes is responsible for "sex-linked" medical conditions that pass through some families, such as type-2 diabetes and the blood disorder haemophilia, mainly affecting males.

The mix of approximately thirty thousand genes present on chromosomes will determine the following:

- the colour of the baby's eyes
- hair
- body shape
- the presence or lack of dimples
- a great singing voice

While thirty thousand genes or more is a lot of material to mix and match, countless combinations are possible, so it's not always easy to predict how the baby will look.

While scientists have investigated whether DNA determines the intelligence of an unborn child, the only conclusion they have reached is that the differences between people on intelligence tests are substantially the result of genetic differences.

So the gift of life your parents gave you is just a starting point, and what they do to nurture your development will influence who you are, your values, your strengths and weaknesses, and your ability to grow and prosper.

What Determines a Person's Health

Not all genetic conditions are passed down from our parents; some gene changes occur before birth and can include the following:

- some cancers
- cystic fibrosis
- high cholesterol
- haemophilia
- muscular dystrophy
- congenital disabilities (for example, spina bifida or a cleft lip).

We have a lot to thank our parents for regarding our genetic makeup. Notably, the role models they are and the examples for us every day in what they do, how they manage to handle or deal with personal relationships, finances, lifestyle, food, alcohol, drugs, and much more strongly influence the person we become.

As the old expression goes, "More is caught than taught".

We are role models for our children and have a tremendous responsibility given the examples we have been to them will influence their children and hopefully the generations that follow.

Jacqui and I had very different backgrounds; I was raised in a working-class family. At the same time, Jacqui's father was a dentist, and her mother was a psychologist. Yet, we hold similar worldviews, work ethics, teaching and learning styles, communication preferences, and lifestyle values that influence a person's health.

Notwithstanding these undeniable facts, generational differences in values, beliefs and opinions will continue to evolve with different generations based on many other events and circumstances due to the changing socioeconomic and cultural changes that influence our world.

The pressure is on each of us to be living, breathing examples to our children and children's children that movement is critical to maintaining a healthy weight, which is essential to a healthy life.

Does Health Determine Fitness or Fitness Health

My life and health struggle overwhelmingly confirm that a person's health is determined by the identity they chose, refined or settled on, and our habits are formed from that identity. I am a living example of how it is possible to change your identity and, in doing so, change the habits that conform to that new identity.

Examples of my new habits:

- I wake to an alarm at 4:30 am seven days a week
- I weigh myself and take note of any changes to my weight
- After getting dressed, I drink a pre-workout supplement
- I walk a minimum of seven kilometres before breakfast
- I listen to audio podcasts, audiobooks and music while I walk
- After breakfast, I shower and get ready for my day
- I read for twenty minutes every morning
- I sit at my desk, and I write in my journal for ten minutes
- I devote two hours to my creative self every day, either writing or painting

My Identity and the habits that support my new identity tell people that "I am a healthy person dedicated to improving the quality of their life and extending their time on this earth".

Genetically, I had all the right gifts: tall, one hundred and ninety-three centimetres, broad-shouldered, physically well-built and proportioned. I had all the strength required, but I never excelled at any sports I played as a teenager and young man.

What I lacked was a role model, that person I wrote about earlier who, through their actions, interactions or observations of me as a young man, could inspire or guide me to be a better person. Had my father been involved in my life and been the inspiration a young man needs, my chances of being a more committed sportsman may have been different.

My father and mother separated when I was twelve, and I had very few male relatives who could fill the role model a father does or other males who influenced my desire to find and maintain the required fitness level to play a higher sports grade.

My father provided me with two genes, ACTN3 and ACE, which influence the fibre type of muscles linked to strength and endurance. The other genes are associated with producing energy for cells, communicating between nerve cells, and functioning skeletal muscles. He failed to provide me with a father's generational obligation to be my mentor, inspiration and role model to his children.

"Even if you can't physically see the result right now, every single effort you make changes your body from the inside. Never get discouraged."

Studies on physical activity and sedentary behaviour adjusted for age, BMI, and educational status confirm a father's sedentary time is significantly associated with boys but not with girls.

The current study results suggest a mother's parental involvement in physical activity is essential for children's physical activity and health outcomes.

Our children and our children's children are our responsibility from a health and fitness perspective. We can institute generational change in health and, as such, the prosperity of our extended and future families.

You need the courage to start!

What's Next

While our genes may have defined who we are, where we come from, and how we grow and learn, it's largely believed the environment we are raised in may influence some of these factors, but how much of an influence science is still debated. While our parent's genes directly influence our development, it's commonly accepted that the child's environment determines how these genes are affected.

Nature or Nurture

We have known for a long time that the mother's genetic makeup has a strong effect on the development of her offspring.

Parents' parenting behaviour must partly genetically determine the influence of transmission. Parents' priorities on reading, sports, health, diet and alcohol and cigarettes are shaped by genes and create a home environment that influences children for better or worse.

So, as a parent, one of the most important decisions you will ever make is to determine what type of example you will be for your children.

Pregnancy

Pregnancy is a turning point in every woman's life, whether planned or unplanned.

No matter what a man reads, hears, or sees, it will never allow him to fully comprehend the emotion associated with a life form starting in a woman's womb. Chromosome contributions aside, to have a life form start, grow and be supported by the mother's body for nine months and then experience childbirth must generate a connection between mother and child no man will ever fully understand.

Two of our three daughters were planned, while the youngest was a mystery. Paige was conceived at the wrong time of the month and against all odds, but she has proven to be a true gift from God to both of us.

I know from Jacqui's perspective that it meant three children under three, which concerned her greatly. While we reconciled the gift we were granted against all odds, it also required significant change, more so for Jacqui than me, but it changed nonetheless.

Jacqui needed to know that I would do whatever was required to help her, and while I knew she was an amazingly strong person, I could see she struggled with the knowledge of what this would need from her.

As for me, the words of support came quickly, but my ability to provide the physical and mental support Jacqui required was much more challenging than the words of assurance I offered.

Jacqui was looking for not words of assurance but the commitment to share the responsibility of raising our three daughters by being there when she needed me or a break from being a mother and a wife. She required me to spend time with her and assume greater responsibility for caring for our daughters.

From my perspective, I had no difficulty spending time at work. That time and effort achieved significant recognition and, in turn, promotion and a requirement to invest more time into my job.

I failed my wife in so many ways. Not deliberately, but I believe it because I came from a generation where the men went to work, and the wife stayed home and raised the children.

Jacqui is perhaps one of the most brilliant marketing people I have ever met. Her ability to quickly see what could be achieved and map out a process to achieve the required outcome is exceptional.

So here she was with three young girls, caring for them and then caring for me at the end of my day.

I failed to recognise that as a brilliant person who no longer had exposure to other people or the opportunities to use her marketing skills, she was isolated and struggled to cope.

I failed my daughters because I did not spend the time with them I could have, and while I am filled with regrets for that failure, I also have to acknowledge that my failure on this front was a direct result of my father's failure to spend time with me.

Habits are learnt from our parents and passed on to future generations.

My gift to you is the wisdom of hindsight.

I chose to follow the lessons from my father when I should have spent more of my time investing in my family.

So, if you are a parent, you need to start parenting your children and partnering with your spouse to ensure you get your children off to the best start possible. It starts with you and the example you set, and you should not be influenced by the standards set by either or both of your parents but by the standard you want to control your patriarchal family.

I recently read the last words Steve Jobs, Apple INC Founder, spoke, and I thought them provocative enough to include them here. The following is not the final transcript; the section deals with the content relevant to the family.

"Therefore, I hope you realise when you have friends, brothers and sisters, with whom you discuss, laugh, talk, sing, talk about north-south-east or heaven and earth, this is the real happiness!

An indisputable fact of life:

"Don't raise your children to be rich. Educate them to be happy. When they grow up, they will know the value of things, not the price."

– Steve Jobs

Educating your children to be happy and know the value of things, not their price, requires you as a parent to focus from the very beginning on the responsibilities of being a parent, which starts for a woman with your health during pregnancy.

Exercise

Moderate aerobic activity during pregnancy of at least hundred fifty minutes every week is considered critical to the health of an unborn baby.

After evaluation by obstetrician-gynaecologists, women with uncomplicated pregnancies can engage in aerobic and strength-conditioning exercises during pregnancy. While this may not have been part of your lifestyle and fitness regime, this is the ideal time to break the habits of a lifetime and start changing what needs to change.

Habits are the most challenging things in the world to break!

Essential Vitamins and Minerals in Pregnancy

Nine months of nourishing your body and a baby's growing body are essential to ensure you eat the right foods and take the supplements required to nurture, and sustain both mother and baby.

Egg yolks are full of choline, a recommended vitamin for pregnant women, which has been shown to improve learning and memory in babies during pregnancy.

Good nutrition in pregnancy is vital for your baby's healthy growth and development. You need to consume enough nutrients to meet your baby's needs and your own.

When pregnant, you need more nutrients, including protein, folate, iodine, iron and some vitamins.

- Folate (called "folic acid" in supplement form) helps prevent neural tube defects, such as spina bifida. When taken at least one month before conception and throughout the first three months of pregnancy
- Iodine is needed for brain and nervous system development
- Iron helps prevent anaemia in the mother, as well as low birth weight in the baby

Vitamin B12 and D are also vital since they support the development of the baby's nervous system (B12) and skeleton (D). Adequate vitamin C intake also helps improve iron absorption from your diet.

DHA, an omega-3 fatty acid, is also associated with better brain development. DHA can be found in many prenatal supplements, but you can also get it by including fish like salmon and sardines in your diet.

Supplements played a vital role in helping me overcome the debilitating effects of so many medical issues. Had I not taken them regularly, my journey to recovery would not have been possible.

Know Your Children Before Their Birth

Studies have shown that parents who talk and read to their babies throughout pregnancy promote early word recognition after birth.

Babies also can recognise the voice and engage with you, and it's an extraordinary time to bond with your child.

Quality Sleep

Getting the right amount of quality sleep is incredibly important. Sleep will help improve your mood, strengthen your immune system, and increase your chances of a healthy birth.

With the right amount of sleep, your baby's brain will have time to develop in the womb while the risk for post-birth developmental issues is significantly reduced.

Sleep During the First Trimester

The main issue in the first trimester is tiredness and the fact that you might also need to pass urine more often, disturbing your sleep.

Sleep During the Second Trimester

The second trimester brings new challenges.

Leg cramps can also disrupt your sleep. It's not understood why leg cramps happen, but you can do several things to ease them, such as stretching your calf muscles, being active during the day and drinking plenty of fluids.

Some women have more dreams than they typically have nightmares. Sometimes, these dreams can be related to stress or inconsistent sleep. If you have dreams disturbing you, it can help to talk to your partner or a friend or consider talking to a counsellor. A regular schedule and maybe try different sleep positions or use a pregnancy pillow.

Sleep During the Third Trimester

You must sleep on your side from twenty-eight weeks till your baby is born. Whether taking a quick nap on the couch or going to bed at night, sleeping on your side is best.

Lying on your back puts pressure on major blood vessels, reducing the blood flow to your womb and restricting your baby's oxygen supply. Research has shown that sleeping on your side can reduce the risk of stillbirth by half.

You can make it more comfortable and easier to stay on your side by bending your knees and putting a pillow between them. You can also set a pillow under your belly for support.

If you wake and find you've been asleep on your back, turn onto your side. If it happens often, put a pillow behind your back so rolling over onto your back is harder.

Avoid heavy lifting, housework and long periods of standing and, as mentioned before, rest during the day with your legs up whenever possible.

The baby might be pressing on your bladder, and the hormones that go with the later stages of pregnancy can relax your pelvic floor. The frequency of your need to pass urine at night might increase even further. Pelvic floor exercises will help you manage any "leaks" and avoid continence problems in years to come.

So here is my gift to you!

Go into your bedroom, strip down your underwear, and look at yourself. If you are unhappy with what you see, ask yourself what needs to change.

If you cannot see the person, you want your children to be when they reach your age. Remember, it is never too late to begin reclaiming your health; I started when I was seventy-two, and while I had to work hard to achieve the health that eluded me for a long, it was worth the cost and effort.

Open your fridge and pantry door, see what you have in these storage areas, and ask yourself, is this the food and drinks I want my children to consume? What will you do if you don't like what you see?

Finally, I want you to start looking at the mixture of food and drink you are consuming as a family, and if it's not as per the mix I have shared with you in Chapter 7, what will you do about that?

It's time to make some decisions because I didn't write this book and spend my time and energy developing the content on my website or recording the thousands of sixty-second messages for people's amusement. I did it because I want you to wake up and that you are probably slowly killing yourself with lousy health choices, just like I did.

Please, get off your ass, and clean the fridge and pantry of all the rubbish you have been eating. Get rid of all the sugar and the products riddled with sugar or sugar substitutes, go to the shops, and restock your food cellar with fresh, healthy food.

Make the lifestyle changes you need to make because if you don't, your health will make them for you.

Live a great life, and enjoy your children and grandchildren. They are the most incredible creations you will ever make, but only possible if you choose health instead of living with the habits that will kill you unless you change them.

To the Fathers

If your father were the role model we all wanted to have as a father, that would be fantastic; you have all you need. If he was not the perfect role model, then you need to ask yourself what changes you need to make to do the best job of helping your children find the health, wealth and happiness we all need and want.

Importantly, it means not spending more time at work. It's spending quality time with your wife and children. It is by spending time one-on-one with them and talking, listening, and making the changes you need to make. It is all about being the father they need, and the only way you will ever know what that need is.

Summary

We had no say in the conception process; we are byproducts of an act of sex, no different to every other reproductive system in the universe. For the great majority, we are cared for and loved by one or more parents who sometimes never planned for our existence and certainly never consider the lifestyle changes that would be forced upon them as a consequence of that act of intimacy.

Gifts are often well-received, sometimes received but never used and sometimes rejected, but we have no choice with what is gifted. None of us came with a user manual. We just got on with living the life our parents gave us. Still, the compound effect of years of poor lifestyle habits will rob us of the quality of life we are entitled to experience and could have if we only made better choices or were prepared to reclaim our health.

Importantly, what we do with the gift makes us unique.

We are all born with the skills required to change our lives, minds, bodies, future, prosperity, and, indeed, our universe. What we are not all born with is equality. Where we are born, who our parents are, and the socioeconomics of the environment we are raised in all influence who we are and the life we will live.

This week, I read a story about a young girl raised in the slums of Calcutta who became the FIDE Women's Rapid Chess Champion at 15 and went on to win the title of the youngest-ever chess grandmaster. This young woman was gifted with no advantages. One might argue that the reverse was that she was numerously disadvantaged but rose above all adversity with determination.

Life can be whatever you want it to be; you can let poor health dictate the quality of your life or take the steps you need to live the life you want to live and be a beacon and a living example for the people you love, who love you, your children, your grandchildren and hundreds of other who will see your health transformation.

"Be the example you need to be."

"Life is the first gift, love is the second, and understanding the third."

– *Marge Piercy*

Chapter 3
Health is a Choice

How do you choose health?

Is that even a possibility?

These fascinating questions can be answered in several different ways.

For healthy people, it is either an active choice or a continuation of a generational health journey started by one or both of their parents.

Alternatively, it may have been a decision to play a particular sport that started you on your fitness journey, culminating in developing healthy habits you maintained throughout your life.

Or could it be simply that poor health brought you to a point where changing the habits of a lifetime was essential for you to live a longer life or a better quality of life?

If it is the latter, then let me tell you that living longer is not a better option; living longer with a better quality of life and a healthier lifestyle filled with energy and passion is unquestionably the best possible outcome.

Being overweight adversely affected my health, resulting in kidney disease, high blood pressure, type-2 diabetes, heart attack, stroke, cardiovascular diseases, prostate cancer, and other minor but debilitating medical problems.

It caused me to fail as the head of my family, placed unnecessary personal and emotional pressure on my wife and daughters and brought me to self-harm and attempted suicide. I had no joy or passion and fell into passive survival.

Health is a choice, and I decided to do whatever it took to improve my health in September 2021 when I chose to stand up and be counted to change the lifestyle habits that dragged me to a point where I was existing. I had to lose the weight that was slowly killing me and reverse all the medical conditions sucking my life force from my body.

The journey was not planned; on the contrary, it started with documenting where I was then, my weight, chest, waist and hip measurements, two photographs, and a statement detailing why I needed to do this and what I hoped to get out of the journey.

Over time, as I started to lose weight, the pain in my legs eased, and my energy levels increased. I found a passion for what I was doing and a hope that, in some way, this health journey of mine might be able to help others. This passion helped me focus on creating sixty-second posts on Instagram. Comments from people following my post encouraged me to believe people were interested in what I was doing and my struggle to overcome my health issues.

This book was a logical extension of what I was doing in my sixty-second posts and a more effective and detailed account of my health journey.

Global Statistics on Obesity

According to WHO (World Health Organisation), worldwide obesity has The Centres for Disease Control and Prevention (CDC), people who are obese, compared to those with a healthy weight, are at increased risk for many severe diseases and health conditions, including the following:

- Heart attack
- High blood pressure (hypertension)
- High LDL cholesterol, low HDL cholesterol, or high levels of triglycerides (Dyslipidemia)
- Type-2 diabetes
- Coronary heart disease
- Stroke
- Gallbladder disease
- Osteoarthritis (a breakdown of cartilage and bone within a joint)
- Sleep apnoea and breathing problems
- Many types of cancers
- Low quality of life
- Mental illnesses such as clinical depression, anxiety, and other mental disorders
- Body pain and difficulty with physical functioning

While reaching and maintaining a healthy weight is good for your overall health, it also reduces the risk of developing any medical conditions listed above. So if Health is a choice and maintaining a healthy weight has the added benefit of helping you feel good about yourself and having more energy to enjoy life, why is it so hard to make that choice?

I believe the answer is as simple as *habits*.

Old habits are hard to break, and new ones are even harder to establish, particularly if they conflict with the old ones.

A person's ideal body weight results from many things: height, genes, metabolism, behaviour, environment and the lifestyle habits they formed. Maintaining a healthy weight requires the correct mix of carbohydrates, proteins, and fats (energy IN) relative to being physically active (energy OUT).

Our choices concerning health start at a very early age; more often than not, we begin by following the examples set by our parents, and those examples become habits.

The old expression that more is caught than taught holds a lot of water in this argument, given we model ourselves on our parents, what they do, what they eat, drink, exercise, what sports they play, and so on.

So it should be no surprise when we see adults who are overweight that their children are similarly overweight.

I have never met anyone who wanted to be overweight, a sumo wrestler, perhaps; I have, however, met a lot of people who were overweight (according to statistics, six out of every ten people are overweight) who wanted to lose weight but either didn't know how to do it or if they found a way we're unable to maintain their new lower weight.

Poor habits over time cause weight gain, and the ability to change those habits by creating new neural pathways (habits) that replace the old neural pathways will always be challenging. So the big question is, how do I change those habits and make them part of my new identity?

Some people believe willpower is the answer, that willpower can overcome almost any temptation.

Willpower

Willpower doesn't work; if it did, you would be slim, healthy, fabulous, wealthy, have everything you ever wanted, and wouldn't be reading this book.

Goals

Set realistic goals and devise a plan to help you achieve them, or the experts tell you. The only problem with goals is they are a final destination, a measurable end position and as such, once reached, what do you do next?

Identity

In his book *7 Habits of Highly Effective People*, Stephen Covey described a hypothetical situation where he woke one morning and was greeted by a stranger waiting to drive him to an appointment. No words were spoken. He just felt compelled to get into the car. The car stopped at a nearby church, and as he walked into the church, he saw several people he knew and loved. At that point, he realised he was attending his funeral; a friend of Stephen's was waiting to deliver Stephen's eulogy. What would his friend say?

Covey promotes a reality most of us have never contemplated; he wrote, what would your best friend say if you could write the eulogy he was about to deliver?

If you look at Covey's story as an opportunity to write your eulogy, what would you have your best friend say about you?

With this opportunity to rewrite your story, what would you change? What would you do differently? Would you define the legacy you want to leave behind and articulate your passion for life, family, and friends?

If you were allowed to rewrite your history, you would change your identity. Habits define an identity, habits others would admire and desire to emulate.

Health Risks Linked to Excess Weight and Obesity

Excess weight, especially obesity, diminishes almost every aspect of health, from reproductive and respiratory function to memory and mood. Obesity increases the risk of several debilitating and deadly diseases, including diabetes, heart disease, and some cancers. It does this in various ways, some as straightforward as the mechanical stress of carrying extra kilograms and some involving complex changes in hormones and metabolism. Obesity decreases the quality and length of life and places unnecessary strain on the family, which becomes collateral damage.

I have provided details of the medical condition affected by being overweight and obese so you can fully understand the consequences of your choices and the habits you may have allowed to influence the quality of life you were designed to experience.

Health is a word invented to describe a general sense of well-being and, as such, can not be measured and is, therefore, a fantasy we either embrace or ignore. I have done so because if you are anything like me, you don't believe these medical issues will impact your health. However, the reality is that "from the moment we were born, we start dying".

Ignoring your health will make you realise that your first significant health issue could have been averted had you only made better choices regarding your eating, drinking, exercise and mental health habits.

Take some time to review each medical condition in the following pages and look carefully at the warning signs associated with each situation. The probability that you are already experiencing some of these signs is a reality that may help you make the decision that will help you reclaim your health and start living the quality of life you were designed to live.

Heart Attack

A heart attack occurs when a coronary artery, which supplies blood to your heart, becomes blocked. The most common sign of an attack is chest discomfort or pain, spreading to your arms, neck, jaw, or back.

Chest discomfort or pain can last for several minutes or come and go.

Risk factors include:

1. Age. Men aged forty-five or older and women aged fifty-five or older are more likely to have an attack than younger men and women.
2. Tobacco. Including smoking and long-term exposure to secondhand smoke.
3. *High blood pressure.* High blood pressure that occurs with other conditions, such as *obesity, high cholesterol* or *diabetes*, increases your risk. Over time, high blood pressure can damage arteries that lead to your heart.
4. Metabolic syndrome. This syndrome occurs when you have *obesity, high blood pressure* and *high blood sugar*. Having metabolic syndrome makes you twice as likely to develop *heart disease* as if you don't.
5. *High blood cholesterol* or *triglyceride levels*. A high level of low-density lipoprotein (LDL) cholesterol ("bad" cholesterol) is most likely to

narrow arteries. However, a high level of high-density lipoprotein (HDL) cholesterol ("good" cholesterol) may lower your risk. A high level of triglycerides, a type of *blood fat related to your diet*, also increases your risk of a heart attack.

6. Obesity. *Obesity* is linked with *high blood cholesterol, triglyceride, blood pressure*, and *diabetes*. Losing just 10% of your body weight can lower this risk.

7. Diabetes. Not producing enough of a hormone secreted by your pancreas (insulin) or not responding to insulin causes your body's blood sugar levels to rise, increasing your risk of a heart attack.

8. Family history of heart attacks. If your siblings, parents or grandparents have had early heart attacks (by age fifty-five for males and sixty-five for females), you might be at increased risk.

9. *Lack of physical activity.* Being inactive contributes to high blood cholesterol levels and obesity. People who exercise regularly have better heart health, including lower blood pressure.

10. Stress. You might respond to stress in ways that can increase your risk of a heart attack.

11. An autoimmune condition. A disease such as rheumatoid arthritis or lupus can increase your risk of a heart attack.

A heart attack requires emergency treatment to restore blood flow to your heart.

Always call Triple Zero (000) immediately if you think you or someone else may have a heart attack.

The most common cause of a heart attack is coronary heart disease, which occurs when the coronary artery, which supplies blood to your heart, narrows because of plaque build-up. Plaque is made of fat, cholesterol, and other materials. The narrowed artery causes a reduced amount of blood flow to your heart muscle.

During a heart attack, plaque from the artery wall breaks away (ruptures) and can form a clot, block blood flow through the artery and cause damage to the heart muscle.

A great resource to gain information about heart attacks is the Australian Heart Foundation.

Get the picture.

High Blood Pressure

What is Hypertension or High Blood Pressure? It is when your blood pressure increases to unhealthy levels.

Your blood pressure measurement considers how much blood passes through your blood vessels and the amount of resistance the blood meets while pumping.

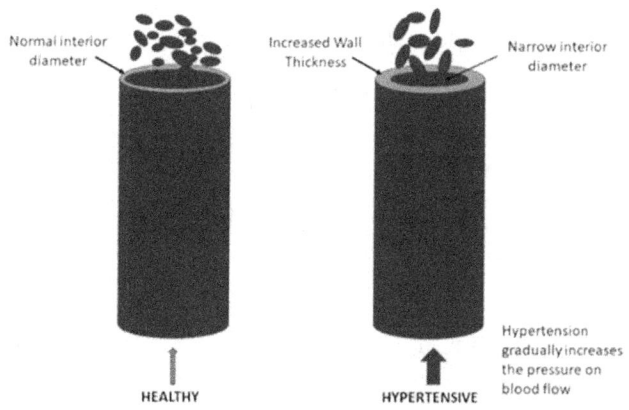

Normal interior diameter

Increased Wall Thickness

Narrow interior diameter

Hypertension gradually increases the pressure on blood flow

HEALTHY   **HYPERTENSIVE**

Narrow arteries increase resistance. The narrower your arteries are, the higher your blood pressure will be. Over the long term, any increase in your blood pressure can cause health issues, including heart disease.

Hypertension is quite common, with one in every four men and one in every five women in Australia suffering from high blood pressure.

Hypertension typically develops over several years. Usually, you don't notice any symptoms. But even without symptoms, *high blood pressure can cause damage to* your *blood vessels* and *organs*, especially the *brain, heart, eyes,* and *kidneys*.

Early detection is essential. Regular blood pressure readings help you and your doctor notice any changes. If your blood pressure is elevated, your doctor may have you check your blood pressure over a few weeks to see if the number stays elevated or falls back to normal levels.

Treatment for hypertension includes both prescription medication and healthy lifestyle changes. If the condition isn't treated, it could lead to health issues, including heart attack and stroke.

What Causes High Blood Pressure?

For most adults, there's no identifiable cause of high blood pressure. This type of high blood pressure, called primary (essential) hypertension, tends to develop gradually over many years.

Some people have high blood pressure caused by an underlying condition. This type of high blood pressure, called secondary hypertension, tends to appear suddenly and cause higher blood pressure than primary hypertension. Various conditions and medications can lead to secondary hypertension, including:

- Obstructive sleep apnoea
- Kidney disease
- Adrenal gland tumours
- Thyroid problems
- Certain defects you're born with (congenital) in blood vessels

Certain medications, such as birth control pills, cold remedies, decongestants, over-the-counter pain relievers and some prescription drugs and illegal drugs, such as cocaine and amphetamines.

Primary Hypertension

Primary hypertension is also called essential hypertension. Most people have this type of high blood pressure. This kind of hypertension develops over time with no identifiable cause.

Researchers are still unclear about what mechanisms cause blood pressure to increase slowly. A combination of factors may play a role. These factors include:

Secondary Hypertension

Secondary hypertension often occurs quickly and can become more severe than primary hypertension. Several conditions that may cause secondary hypertension include:

- kidney disease
- obstructive sleep apnoea
- congenital heart defects
- problems with your thyroid
- side effects of medications
- use of illegal drugs
- alcohol abuse or chronic use
- adrenal gland problems
- certain endocrine tumours

What are the Symptoms of Hypertension?

Hypertension is called a "silent killer". Most people with hypertension are unaware of the problem because it may have no warning signs or symptoms. For this reason, blood pressure must be measured regularly.

They can include early morning headaches, nosebleeds, irregular heart rhythms, vision changes, and ear buzzing when symptoms occur. Severe hypertension can cause fatigue, nausea, vomiting, confusion, anxiety, chest pain, and muscle tremors.

The only way to detect hypertension is to have a health professional measure blood pressure. Having blood pressure measured is quick and painless. Although individuals can measure their blood pressure using automated devices, an evaluation by a health professional is essential for assessing risk and associated conditions.

High LDL Cholesterol, Low HDL Cholesterol, High Levels of Triglycerides

Two types of lipoproteins carry cholesterol to and from cells. The first lipoprotein is low-density (LDL). The other is high-density lipoprotein (HDL).

LDL (Bad) Cholesterol

LDL cholesterol is considered the "bad" cholesterol because it contributes to fatty buildups in arteries, which causes narrowing of the arteries and increases the risk for heart attack, stroke and peripheral artery disease.

HDL (Good) Cholesterol

HDL cholesterol can be considered "good" because a healthy level may protect against heart attack and stroke.

HDL carries LDL cholesterol from the arteries and back to the liver, where the LDL is broken down and passed from the body. But HDL cholesterol doesn't eliminate LDL cholesterol. HDL carries only one-third to one-fourth of blood cholesterol.

Lipoprotein(a), or Lp(a) Cholesterol

Unlike the other types of bad cholesterol, LDL, Lp(a) is mainly linked to genetics. Elevated Lp(a) among families with a history of heart attacks or people with heart attacks and strokes in their thirties is more common than lifestyle factors.

Lp(a) comprises particles that carry cholesterol around the body and is a significant risk factor for atherosclerosis, which is the hardening and narrowing of the arteries.

Triglycerides

Triglycerides are the most common type of fat in the body. They store excess energy from your diet.

A high triglyceride level combined with high LDL (bad) cholesterol or low HDL (good) cholesterol is linked with fatty buildups within the artery walls, which increases the risk of heart attack and stroke.

Type-2 Diabetes

Type-2 diabetes, formerly known as adult-onset diabetes, is a form of diabetes characterised by high blood sugar, insulin resistance, and a relative lack of insulin. Common symptoms include increased thirst, frequent urination, and unexplained weight loss.

Long-term complications from high blood sugar include heart disease, strokes, diabetic retinopathy, blindness, kidney failure, and poor blood flow in the limbs, leading to amputations. Symptoms may also include increased hunger, tiredness, and sores that do not heal. Often, symptoms come on slowly.

The sudden onset of a hyperosmolar hyperglycemic state may occur; however, ketoacidosis is uncommon.

Type 2 diabetes primarily occurs due to *obesity* and *lack of exercise.* Some people are more genetically at risk than others.

Type-2 diabetes makes up about 90% of cases of diabetes, with the other 10% due primarily to type-1 diabetes and gestational diabetes.

In Type-1 diabetes, there is a lower total level of insulin to control blood glucose due to an autoimmune-induced loss of insulin-producing beta cells in the pancreas.

Diagnosis of diabetes is by blood tests such as fasting plasma glucose, oral glucose tolerance test, or glycated haemoglobin.

Type 2 diabetes is largely preventable by staying within an average weight range, *exercising regularly,* and *eating a healthy diet* (high in fruits and vegetables and low in sugar and saturated fats).

Treatment involves *exercise* and *dietary changes.* Metformin is typically recommended if blood sugar levels are not adequately lowered. Many people may eventually also require insulin injections.

Routinely checking blood sugar levels in those on insulin is advised; however, this may not be needed in those taking pills. Bariatric surgery often improves diabetes in those who are *obese.*

Coronary Heart Disease

Coronary heart disease (CHD) is Australia's single leading cause of disease burden and death. There are two primary clinical forms—heart attack (also known as acute myocardial infarction) and angina. A heart attack is life-threatening when a blood vessel supplying the heart is blocked entirely. Angina is a chronic condition in which short episodes of chest pain occur periodically when the heart has a temporary deficiency in its blood supply.

CHD is largely preventable, as many of its risk factors are modifiable. These include tobacco smoking, biomedical risk factors such as *high blood pressure* and *high blood cholesterol, insufficient physical activity, poor diet and nutrition, and obesity.* As a result of the substantial burden of CHD on the population, a National Strategic Action Plan for Heart Disease and Stroke is under development. The action plan aims to reflect priorities and identify implementable actions to reduce the impact of CHD in the community.

Stroke

A stroke is a medical emergency. A stroke occurs when the blood supply to a part of your brain is suddenly reduced, preventing that part of your brain from getting oxygen and other nutrients from your blood.

Your brain needs a continuous supply of oxygen and nutrients from the blood your arteries supply. Without oxygen or nutrients, your brain cells will die (infarct), and the affected area can suffer permanent damage.

Two main reasons for reduced blood supply are blood clots and bleeding.

Key Facts

A stroke occurs when your brain can't get enough oxygen and essential nutrients, usually because a blood clot or sudden bleed reduces the blood supply.

Signs of a stroke include a drooping face, difficulty moving your arms, or slurred speech.

If you notice signs of a stroke, call triple zero (000) immediately since any delay may lead to permanent brain damage or death.

You can reduce your chance of stroke by managing risk factors such as *high blood pressure* and *cholesterol*, *eating healthily*, and *exercising*.

Causes of a Stroke

High Blood Pressure

Your doctor may call it hypertension, the most significant cause of strokes. Your doctor will discuss treatments if your blood pressure is typically 140/90 or higher.

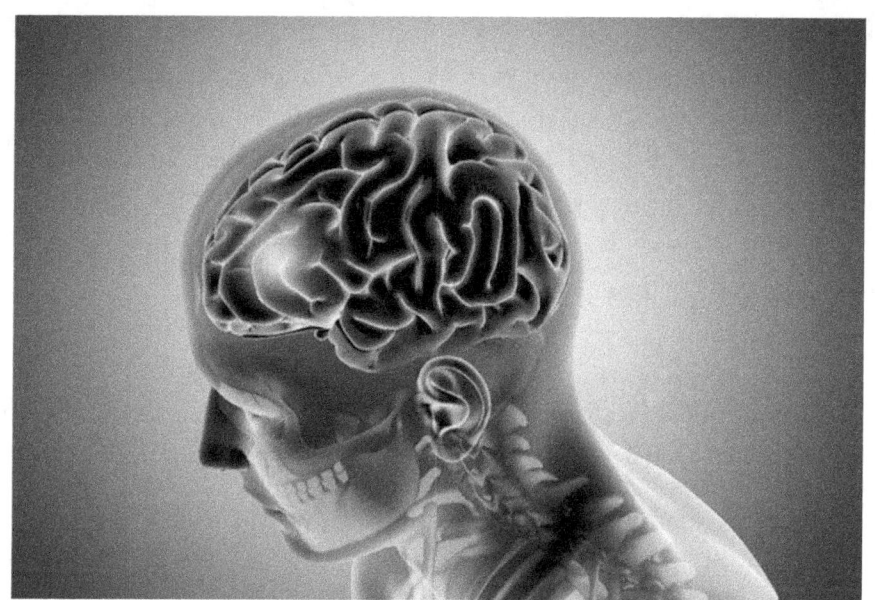

Tobacco

Smoking or chewing it raises your odds of a stroke. Nicotine makes your blood pressure go up. Cigarette smoke causes a fatty build-up in your main neck artery. It also thickens your blood and makes it more likely to clot. Even secondhand smoke can affect you.

Heart Disease

This condition includes defective heart valves and atrial fibrillation, or irregular heartbeat, which causes a quarter of all strokes among older people. You can also have clogged arteries from fatty deposits.

Diabetes

People with diabetes also have *high blood pressure* and are more likely to be *overweight*. Both raise the chance of a stroke. Diabetes damages your blood vessels, which makes a stroke more likely. If you have a stroke when your *blood sugar levels are high*, the injury to your brain is more significant.

Weight and exercise. Your chances of a stroke may go up if you're *overweight*. You can lower your odds by working out every day. Take a *brisk thirty-minute walk*, or do *muscle-strengthening exercises* like pushups and working with weights.

Medications

Some medicines can raise your chances of stroke. For instance, blood-thinning drugs, which doctors suggest to prevent blood clots, can sometimes make a stroke more likely through bleeding. Studies have linked hormone therapy, used for menopause symptoms like hot flashes, with a higher risk of strokes. And low-dose oestrogen in birth control pills may also increase your odds.

Age

Anyone could have a stroke, even babies in the womb. Generally, your chances go up as you get older. They double every decade after the age of fifty-five.

Family

Strokes can run in families. You and your relatives may share a tendency to get *high blood pressure* or *diabetes*. Some strokes can be brought on by a genetic disorder that blocks blood flow to the brain.

Gender

Women are slightly less likely to have a stroke than men of the same age. But women have strokes later, making them less likely to recover and more likely to die.

Race

Strokes affect African Americans and non-white Hispanic Americans much more often than any other group in the US. Sickle cell disease, a genetic condition that can narrow arteries and interrupt blood flow, is also more common in these groups and in people whose families come from the Mediterranean, the Middle East, or Asia.

Gallbladder Disease

https://www.healthline.com/health/gallbladder-disease

The term gallbladder disease is used for several conditions affecting your gallbladder.

The gallbladder is a small pear-shaped sac located underneath your liver. Your gallbladder's primary function is to store the bile produced by your liver and pass it through a duct that empties into the small intestine. Bile helps you digest fats in your small intestine.

Inflammation causes most gallbladder diseases due to irritating the gallbladder walls, known as cholecystitis. This inflammation is often due to gallstones blocking the ducts, leading to the small intestine and causing bile to build up. It may eventually lead to necrosis (tissue destruction) or gangrene.

What are the types of gallbladder disease?

There are many different types of gallbladder disease.

Gallstones

Gallstones develop when substances in the bile (such as cholesterol, bile salts, and calcium) or substances from the blood (like bilirubin) form hard particles that block the passageways to the gallbladder and bile ducts.

Gallstones also form when the gallbladder doesn't empty completely or often enough. They can be as small as a grain of sand or as large as a golf ball.

Numerous factors contribute to your risk of gallstones. These include:

- *being overweight or obese*
- *having diabetes*
- being age sixty or older
- taking medications that contain oestrogen
- having a family history of gallstones
- being female
- having Crohn's disease and other conditions that affect how nutrients are absorbed
- having cirrhosis or other liver diseases

Cholecystitis

Cholecystitis is the most common type of gallbladder disease. It presents itself as either an acute or chronic inflammation of the gallbladder.

Acute cholecystitis:

Gallstones generally cause acute cholecystitis. But it may also be the result of tumours or various other illnesses.

It may present with pain in the upper right side or upper-middle part of the abdomen. The pain occurs right after a meal and ranges from sharp pangs to dull aches that can radiate to your right shoulder. Acute cholecystitis can also cause:

- fever
- nausea
- vomiting
- jaundice
- Chronic cholecystitis

After several attacks of acute cholecystitis, the gallbladder can shrink and lose its ability to store and release bile. Abdominal pain, nausea, and vomiting may occur. Surgery is often the needed treatment for chronic cholecystitis.

Choledocholithiasis

Gallstones may become lodged in the neck of the gallbladder or the bile ducts. When the gallbladder is plugged in, bile can't exit which may lead to the gallbladder becoming inflamed or distended.

The plugged bile ducts prevent bile from travelling from the liver to the intestines. Choledocholithiasis can cause:

- extreme pain in the middle of your upper abdomen
- fever
- chills
- nausea
- vomiting
- jaundice
- pale- or clay-coloured stools

Acalculous Gallbladder Disease

Acalculous gallbladder disease is inflammation of the gallbladder that occurs without gallstones. Having a significant chronic illness or serious medical condition has triggered an episode.

Symptoms are similar to acute cholecystitis with gallstones. Some risk factors for the condition include:

- severe physical trauma
- heart surgery
- abdominal surgery
- severe burns
- autoimmune conditions like lupus
- bloodstream infections
- receiving nutrition intravenously (IV)
- significant bacterial or viral illnesses

Biliary Dyskinesia

Biliary dyskinesia occurs when the gallbladder has a lower-than-normal function. This condition may be related to ongoing gallbladder inflammation.

There are usually no gallstones in the gallbladder with biliary dyskinesia. Symptoms include abdominal pain after eating, nausea, bloating, and indigestion. Eating a fatty meal may trigger symptoms.

Biliary dyskinesia is usually diagnosed if the gallbladder can only release 35% to 40% or less of its contents. Your doctor may need a HIDA scan test to help diagnose this condition. This test measures gallbladder function.

Sclerosing Cholangitis

Ongoing inflammation and damage to the bile duct system can lead to scarring. This condition is referred to as sclerosing cholangitis. However, it's unknown what exactly causes this disease.

Nearly half the people with this condition don't have symptoms. If symptoms do occur, they can include:

- fever
- jaundice
- itching
- upper abdominal discomfort

Approximately 60% to 80% of trusted sources of people with this condition also have ulcerative colitis. Having this condition does increase the risk of liver cancer as well. Currently, the only known cure is a liver transplant.

Medications that suppress the immune system and those that help break down thickened bile can help manage symptoms.

Gallbladder Cancer

Cancer of the gallbladder is a relatively rare disease. There are different types of gallbladder cancers. They can be challenging to treat because they're not often diagnosed until late in the disease's progression. Gallstones are a common risk factor trusted source for gallbladder cancer.

Gallbladder cancer can spread from the inner walls of the gallbladder to the outer layers and then to the liver, lymph nodes, and other organs. The symptoms of gallbladder cancer may be similar to acute cholecystitis, but there may also be no symptoms.

Gallbladder Polyps

Gallbladder polyps are lesions or growths that occur within the gallbladder. They're usually benign and have no symptoms. They have a greater chance of being cancerous. However, removing the gallbladder for polyps larger than one centimetre is often recommended.

Gangrene of the Gallbladder

Gangrene can occur when the gallbladder develops inadequate blood flow and is one of the most severe complications of acute cholecystitis. Factors that increase the risk of this complication include:

- being male and over forty-five years old
- having diabetes

The symptoms of gallbladder gangrene can include the following:

- dull pain in the gallbladder region
- fever
- nausea or vomiting
- disorientation
- low blood pressure
- Abscess of the gallbladder

Abscess of the gallbladder results when the gallbladder becomes inflamed with pus. Pus accumulates white blood cells, dead tissue, and bacteria. Symptoms may include upper right-sided pain in the abdomen, fever, and shaking chills.

This condition can occur during acute cholecystitis when a gallstone blocks the gallbladder completely, allowing the gallbladder to fill with pus. It's more common in people with diabetes and heart disease.

Osteoarthritis

https://www.cdc.gov/arthritis/basics/osteoarthritis.htm

Osteoarthritis (OA) is the most common form of arthritis. Some call it a degenerative joint disease or "wear and tear" arthritis. It occurs most frequently in the hands, hips, and knees.

With OA, the cartilage within a joint begins to break down, and the underlying bone changes. These changes usually develop slowly and get worse over time. OA can cause pain, stiffness, and swelling. It also causes reduced function and disability; some people can no longer do daily tasks or work.

What are the signs and symptoms of OA?
- Pain or aching
- Stiffness
- Decreased range of motion (or flexibility)
- Swelling

What are the risk factors for OA?
- Joint injury or overuse—Injury or overuse, such as knee bending and repetitive stress on a joint, can damage and increase the risk of OA in that joint.
- Age—The risk of developing OA increases with age.
- Gender—Women are more likely to develop OA than men, especially after the age of fifty.
- Obesity—Extra weight stresses joints, particularly weight-bearing joints like the hips and knees. This stress increases the risk of OA in that joint. *Obesity* may also have metabolic effects that increase the risk of OA.

- Genetics—People with OA family members are more likely to develop OA. People who have hand OA are more likely to develop knee OA.
- Race—Some Asian populations have a lower risk for OA.

Sleep Apnea

Sleep Apnea is a medical condition where you repeatedly stop and start breathing while sleeping. It occurs when your throat muscles intermittently relax to collapse, blocking the airway during sleep, often causing the person to snore. There are several types of sleep apnea, but the most common type is obstructive.

The second type is called Central, which occurs when your brain doesn't send proper signals to the muscles that control breathing.

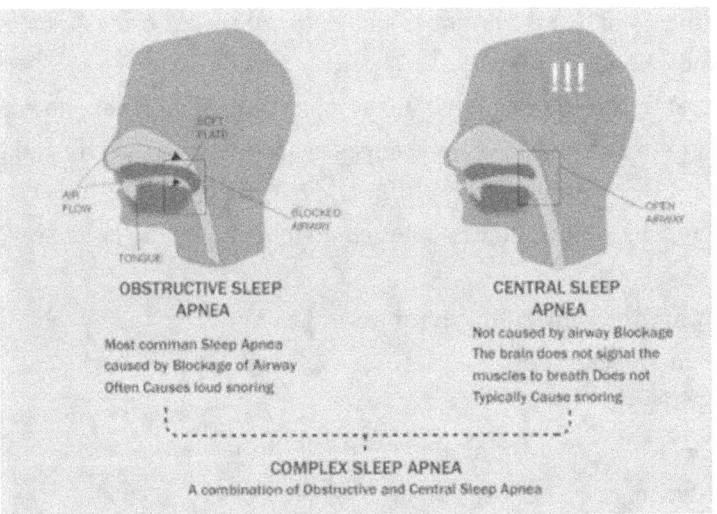

OBSTRUCTIVE SLEEP APNEA

Most common Sleep Apnea caused by Blockage of Airway Often Causes loud snoring

CENTRAL SLEEP APNEA

Not caused by airway Blockage The brain does not signal the muscles to breath Does not Typically Cause snoring

COMPLEX SLEEP APNEA
A combination of Obstructive and Central Sleep Apnea

Only 3% of people in the normal-weight range develop the condition, but the percentage jumps considerably for people who are *overweight or obese to a staggering 20%.*

Sleep Apnea affects men more than women, while the percentage increases sharply in women after menopause.

Sleep Apnea can cause short-term sleep deprivation, affecting mood and safety at work and while driving.

It's also strongly linked to life-threatening chronic conditions like *heart disease, high blood pressure, stroke, Type-2 diabetes*, and *depression.*

Treatments for Sleep Apnea involve using a device (CPAP) that uses positive pressure to keep your airway open while you sleep.

Symptoms of Sleep Apnoea include:

- Poor quality sleep with regular periods of reduced or absent breathing, often accompanied by loud snoring and gasping for air
- Dry mouth and headaches upon waking
- Daytime sleepiness and fatigue
- Irritability and mood changes
- Poor concentration memory and slow reaction times
- Depression and anxiety
- Impotence (erectile dysfunction) and reduced sex drive (libido)
- The need to get up to the toilet frequently at night

Cancers

Hardly anyone I know has not lost a loved one or friend from this insidious disease. My mother and stepfather were heavy smokers who died from lung cancer, while my only encounter was the surgical removal of several skin cancers.

Low Quality of Life

The relationship between excess weight and psychological well-being is complex, encompassing physical, social and psychological factors. Furthermore, this relationship is bidirectional: living with obesity impairs quality of life and increases the risk of psychiatric and affective disorders; conversely, patients with psychological troubles may become *obese* as a medication side effect and use food as a coping strategy.

Many individuals living with *obesity* experience self-blame, low self-esteem, and general negativity towards themselves and their situation. Managing obesity-related distress can directly improve QoL and indirectly affect health behaviours such as treatment adherence. For this reason, distress should not be regarded as a mental health matter but as a *critical factor in successful long-term weight management.*

Mental Illness (Depression)

Depression is a common illness worldwide, affecting an estimated 4% of the population.

Approximately 290 million people in the world have or have experienced depression.

Depression is different from what may be labelled as mood fluctuations or short-lived emotional responses to challenges in everyday life.

It can cause the affected person to function poorly at work, at school and in the family and can lead to more severe health conditions and it can lead to suicide.

It is estimated that somewhere between 700,000 and 800,000 people die yearly from suicide.

Suicide is the fourth leading cause of death in fifteen to twenty-nine-year-olds who may become seriously ill.

Although there are known, effective treatments for mental disorders, 75% of low- to middle-income countries receive no treatment.

Barriers to effective care include a lack of trained healthcare providers and the social stigma associated with mental disorders.

The Black Dog Institute was established in 1985 as a charity offering peer-to-peer support for people struggling with mental health.

Consisting of volunteers who have lived experiences of their mental health battles and understand what someone suffering from depression is going through. They offer *free online* support via a chat service every day.

Body Pain and Difficulty with Physical Functioning

Pain is the body's way of drawing your attention to the fact that you should stop doing whatever caused that pain. Pick up a hot pan on the stove, and the body's pain signals to the brain is a simple message: let go of the pan, fool.

But for some, the inability to feel pain can have life-threatening consequences.

The damage to my legs' nerves caused by *type-2 diabetes* means that walking barefoot anywhere is not an option. On one occasion, after standing on a piece of glass, I noticed blood on the while tyles where I stood. I could see the blood train I had left after standing on the glass. I had not felt the glass cut my foot or the pain associated with every step.

Conversely, the nerve pain in my feet at night kept me awake and looking for relief to help overcome the pain and allow me a good night's sleep. Strange that a cut, I failed to register any pain, but the nerve pain was acute and impossible to sleep.

Depending on its severity, pain can physically impair your ability to work, cope, and make the right decisions. Pain, in combination with a lack of quality sleep, can cause you to make life-threatening decisions for yourself and others.

Obesity

Obesity is defined, according to the <u>World Health Organisation,</u> as abnormal or excessive fat accumulation that presents a health risk. A body mass index (BMI) over 25 is considered overweight, and over 30 is obese.

According to the global disease burden, the issue has grown to epidemic proportions, with *over 4 million deaths yearly due to being overweight or obese in 2017.*

About three-quarters (74.5%) of Australian men were overweight or obese, compared with 59.7% of women.

Statistics show that 42% of men and 29.6% of women were overweight but not obese.

While 32.5% of men and 30.2% of women were obese.

While BMI (Body Mass Index) is an internationally recognised measurement of obesity, other measurements are equally accepted.

Waist Circumference

The National Heart, Lung, and Blood Institute recommends that your waist circumference be less than 101.6cm or 40 inches for men and less than 88.9cm or 35 inches for women.

Waist-to-Height Ratio

A waist-to-height ratio of more than 0.5 may increase your heart disease and diabetes risk.

The World Health Organisation categorises high risk as above 0.85 for women and more than 0.9 for men. You can calculate your waist-to-hip ratio by taking your waist circumference and dividing it by your hip circumference.

Body Fat Percentage

We use the OMRON HBF-514C Full Body Composition Monitor and Scale to calculate BMI, incorporating waist, hips, and chest circumferences to gain the best possible measurement.

Visceral Fat

Visceral fat is a type of body fat stored within the abdominal cavity. It's located near several vital organs, including the liver, stomach, and intestines, and can also build up in the arteries.

Visceral fat is called "active fat" because it can increase the risk of severe health problems.

Kidney Disease

Kidney disease is a general term for when the kidneys are damaged and do not function as they should. If you have kidney disease that lasts for more than three months, it is called chronic kidney disease (or CKD).

Chronic kidney disease involves a gradual loss of kidney function: your kidneys filter wastes and excess fluids from your blood, which are removed when you urinate. When fluid levels, electrolytes and wastes build up in your body because your kidney is not functioning correctly, your medical condition is called Advanced Chronic Kidney Disease, requires dialysis, and if untreated, can cause death.

As kidney disease progresses, you may start feeling unwell. Symptoms of the middle and late stages include:

- high blood pressure
- changes in the amount and number of times you pass urine, such as waking up in the night to urinate
- changes in how the urine looks (such as frothy or foaming urine)
- blood in the urine
- puffiness in the legs, ankles or around the eyes
- pain in the kidney area
- tiredness, lethargy
- loss of appetite
- headaches
- nausea and vomiting
- bad breath and a metallic taste in the mouth
- muscle cramps
- generally feeling unwell

Prostate Cancer

Prostate cancer develops when abnormal cells in the prostate gland grow uncontrollably, forming a malignant tumour.

Prostate cancer is the second most common cancer diagnosed in men in Australia and the third most common cause of cancer death. It is more common in older men, with over 63% of cases diagnosed in men over sixty-five. It is estimated that 18,110 new cases of prostate cancer will be diagnosed in Australia in 2021, while one in six men will be diagnosed with prostate cancer by eighty-five.

Early (localised) prostate cancer refers to cancer cells that have grown but do not appear to have spread beyond the prostate.

There are two stages of advanced prostate cancer:

- locally advanced prostate cancer, where cancer has spread outside the prostate to nearby parts of the body or glands close to the prostate
- metastatic prostate cancer, where cancer has spread to distant parts of the body.

The five-year survival rate for prostate cancer is 95%.

Symptoms

Early prostate cancer usually does not cause symptoms.

Advanced prostate cancer symptoms can include:

- Frequent urination
- Weak or interrupted urine flow or the need to strain to empty the bladder
- The urge to urinate frequently at night
- Blood in the urine
- New onset of erectile dysfunction
- Pain or burning during urination is much less common.

Causes

It's not clear what causes prostate cancer.

Doctors know that prostate cancer begins when cells in the prostate develop changes in their DNA. A cell's DNA contains the instructions that tell a cell what to do and what causes the cells to grow and divide more rapidly than normal cells. The abnormal cells continue living when other cells die.

The accumulating abnormal cells form a tumour that can grow to invade nearby tissue. In time, some abnormal cells can break away and spread (metastasise) to other body parts.

PSA Blood Test

Prostate-specific antigen, or PSA, is a protein normal and malignant prostate gland cells produce. The PSA test measures the level of PSA in the blood. A blood sample is sent to a laboratory for this test for analysis. The results are usually reported as nanograms of PSA per millilitre (ng/mL) of blood.

The blood level of PSA is often elevated in people with prostate cancer. The FDA initially approved the PSA test in 1986 to monitor prostate cancer progression in men who had already been diagnosed with the disease. In 1994, the FDA approved the PSA test for a digital rectal exam (DRE) to detect prostate cancer in men aged fifty and older. Until 2008, many doctors and professional organisations had encouraged yearly PSA screening for prostate cancer beginning at the age of fifty.

PSA testing (along with a DRE) is also often used by healthcare providers for individuals who report prostate symptoms to help determine the nature of the problem.

In addition to prostate cancer, several benign (not cancerous) conditions can cause a person's PSA level to rise, particularly prostatitis (inflammation of the prostate) and benign prostatic hyperplasia (BPH) (enlargement of the prostate). There is no evidence that either condition leads to prostate cancer, but someone can have one or both and develop prostate cancer.

PSA Rising Quickly

The yearly increase in the PSA level is known as the PSA velocity. It is one measure of prostate cancer risk since PSA levels can rise rapidly in men with prostate cancer. It can be beneficial for finding prostate cancer early before it has left the prostate capsule.

Research shows that a yearly increase of.75 ng/mL indicates prostate cancer if a man has a total PSA result between 4.0 and 10.0 ng/mL. Further, a 2.0 ng/mL increase over a year predicts a higher likelihood of death due to aggressive prostate cancer.

Below is a list of the ng/mL ranges for the various ages.

Age	Range
40-49	0-2.5 ng/mL
50-59	0-3.5 ng/mL
60-69	0-4.5 ng/mL
70-79	0-6.5 ng/mL

Digital Rectal Examination

Digital Rectal Examination (DRE) is no longer recommended as a routine test for men without prostate cancer symptoms. Not all prostate cancers produce high levels of PSA, so it may be used to check the prostate before a biopsy.

Biopsy

A biopsy removes small pieces of tissue from different prostate parts with a rectal ultrasound for examination under a microscope. It is used to detect the disease and determine its aggressiveness (the Gleason score of 1-5 is added from two samples to form a score of 10; low scores of 6 or less indicate a slow-growing disease).

Further Tests

If cancer is detected in your prostate, you may have other tests such as MRI, PET, CT, or bone scans to see if the disease is contained in the prostate or help with management and treatment options.

Male Reproductive System and the Prostate

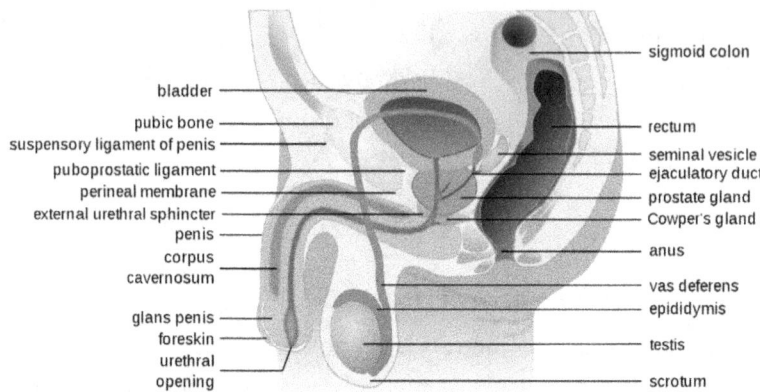

Labels (left side): bladder, pubic bone, suspensory ligament of penis, puboprostatic ligament, perineal membrane, external urethral sphincter, penis, corpus cavernosum, glans penis, foreskin, urethral opening

Labels (right side): sigmoid colon, rectum, seminal vesicle, ejaculatory duct, prostate gland, Cowper's gland, anus, vas deferens, epididymis, testis, scrotum

The prostate is a male reproductive system gland between the bladder and penis.

The urethra is a tube connected to the bladder and the penis, which allows us to pass urine.

The prostate houses a connection to the urethra of the ejaculatory duct vas deferens and the seminal vesicle, through which semen from the testicles mixes with seminal fluid and passes into the urethra as ejaculation.

During a radical prostatectomy, a surgeon removes the entire prostate gland and may also remove tissues around your prostate that include seminal vesicles and lymph nodes used by the body to help fight infection.

Radical prostatectomy is generally very safe. Surgeons protect the nerves that run from the prostate to the penis. However problems due to nerve damage can occur. There is a risk that you may experience:

Urinary Incontinence

Some people experience urinary incontinence, although most people recover continence. Your provider can help you manage the loss of bladder control and urine leakage.

Erectile Dysfunction

Many people have problems maintaining erections after this surgery. The likelihood of recovery of erectile function depends on your erections before surgery and your surgeon's ability to spare the nerves that control erection at the time of surgery.

Choose It or Lose It

As a sales manager, I used this expression to try and convince my salespeople that they needed to use God's gifts more effectively, so I would quote the following.

'God gave you two ears and one mouth; use them directly proportional to God's gift.' Translated, I encouraged them to ask questions, and from the answers would always come more questions. It was always about getting the customer to tell us everything we needed to know to provide the solution suited to their requirements.

Knowing what a person wants and sometimes needs can only come from asking the right questions, and if they don't know what, they need to guide them to the point of clarity. Pushing the solution you want to provide before understanding the person's needs will always fail.

Listening is a skill; hearing what you have been told and using that knowledge to guide a person is the best result you can achieve from using that skill.

Don't just hear what you want; listen to what you need to hear and act on that knowledge.

During World War I, the communication line between the command centre and the front line was cut, so the word was passed down the line, "Send reinforcements; we are going to advance", but the time it had passed through over a hundred soldiers, the message said, "send three and fourpence we are going to a dance".

While all of the above is true from a sales perspective, how does it relate to your health?

Simple, your health, like your ears and your mouth, was a gift from God, and you can accept what you have been given, take it for granted and possibly abuse it in some instances. The one thing I can guarantee is that as sure as your body ages, so does the quality of your health deteriorate, and if you ignore the warning signs and continue to think you are indestructible, then, like me, your health will bite you in the ass.

When you sit with your doctor, don't just accept what you are being told ask questions; it's your health, and if you don't take ownership of your health and make the required changes to your lifestyle, it will be much harder, sometimes impossible, to adjust further down the line.

If you ignore it, you will lose it.

Knowledge is everything, so the art of acquiring that knowledge is just as important as using it to frame the correct response in any situation you can imagine.

If you ignore what I have told you and take the steps required to reclaim your health, you will lose it.

If not your life, you will compromise the quality of your life and have to live with those consequences. Not only that, but your wife, husband, brother, sister, or children will have to deal with your death simply because you heard but didn't listen or act!

Summary

While this list of medical conditions may seem irrelevant to your current health, the various health authorities, including the <u>Australian Institute of Health and Welfare</u>, the <u>World Health Organisation</u>, the <u>Centre for Disease Control and Prevention</u>, and the <u>Mayo Clinic</u>, have confirmed *many of these conditions are caused by being overweight*.

I lived in denial for thirty years that my weight caused any medical problems. As the famous world-renowned philosopher Forrest Gump once said, "Stupid is as Stupid Does".

It's your choice; it's your life, and if you don't believe all that I have outlined in this book, then do your research and speak to your doctor, but please do something because if you don't do something about your health, it will fail you and leave you with nothing but regrets.

Importantly, it will deny you a life filled with love and family, and it will deny family that love and need to spend time with you.

"Time is free, but it's priceless. You can't own it, but you can use it. You can't keep it, but you can spend it. Once you've lost it, you can never get it back."

– Harvey MacKay

"I believe that the greatest gift you can give your family and the world is a healthy you."

– Joyce Meyer

Chapter 4
Choices Have Consequences

Choices have consequences; that is certainly the case with my medical history. All of my medical issues, except Leptospirosis, can be attributed to being overweight. I never thought this was a problem, and while conversations with the various doctors whose care I was under talked about the need to lose a little weight, none of them told me that I would have a heart attack or stroke unless I lost the weight.

My kidneys have been an issue for over twenty years. Until I confronted my doctor recently with the words, "Do I have a significant problem with my kidneys?" did we even talk about how fundamental to my health they were. Fortunately, for the first time, my results from blood taken two days before this conversation were 60 mL/min (Range (>59)), so the doctor's answer was, at the moment, no, you don't have a problem.

I had asked the question because, in writing this book, I collected complete blood and urine test results for over twenty years. When compiling the results, it was apparent that my kidneys were, at one point, Stage 3b kidney disease, and any further decline may have placed me in a position where dialysis was required.

Because the last test result showed an unexplainable improvement, my doctor referred me for an ultrasound of my kidneys.

The ultrasound results came back with evidence of scarring on both kidneys and bilateral renal cysts.

On reviewing the ultrasound results, my doctor was at a loss to explain the dramatic improvement from 46 mL/min to 60 mL/min other than to attribute it to the fact I was consuming more water and had lost a considerable amount of weight.

My latest test results were 67 mL/min, a considerable improvement from my lowest 39 mL/min result.

It is essential to find a doctor you can trust and not just one who treats your conditions systematically by prescribing medications that treat the symptoms while failing to address the cause of the problem. You must also understand that medicine is not a cure for medical issues. But one that allows you to live in denial that the medical problem is something to be concerned about or causes you to adjust to your lifestyle habits.

You can live in denial, or it may be easier to do something about it now and enjoy the life your parents gifted you. I did for many years and worked exceptionally hard to reverse the medical conditions threatening my quality of life.

I chose the hard way; I hope you will learn from my experiences and do it better, do it easier, enjoy life more and be the example to your spouse and children you were always meant to be.

Medical Conditions That Cause Weight Gain

Several medical conditions can cause a person to gain weight, and it is appropriate to include these to ensure we offer a more cognitive and inclusive perspective. Listed below are several conditions doctors believe can cause a person to gain weight apart from the obvious sedimentary issues or poor choices with lifestyle habits.

- Hypothyroidism
- Cushing's Syndrome
- Menopause
- Polycystic Ovary Syndrome
- Depression
- Congestive Heart Failure
- Narcolepsy

Health Effects of Being Overweight or Obese

Let's start with the elephant in the room: obesity.

All my life, I refused to accept that I was obese. Instead, I justified my position by being tall and heavyset, with broad shoulders and a large physical frame and bone structure, or anything else I could use to avoid being placed in that category.

The truth is, I was obese; why? Because my waist measurement was above 100cm and closer to 133cm, the thought of having to consider for a moment that I was obese was just not something I would consider.

The effects of being overweight or obese are significant, so if you think you are overweight or your BMI is higher than 30.0, you risk developing serious complications that will either shorten your life or reduce the quality of your life.

"I know because I lived in denial most of my life. The consequences of that denial have caused me considerable difficulties and more continuous pain than most people would be capable of bearing."

Robert McAnderson

Listed below are the health conditions that can occur due to being overweight. The items shown in red are conditions I have and am currently being treated for.

- High blood pressure (Hypertension)
- High LDL cholesterol, low HDL cholesterol, or high levels of triglycerides (Dyslipidemia)
- Type-1 and 2 diabetes
- Coronary heart disease
- Stroke
- Gallbladder disease
- Kidney disease
- Osteoarthritis (a breakdown of cartilage and bone within a joint)
- Sleep apnoea and breathing problems
- Low quality of life
- Mental illnesses such as clinical depression, anxiety, and other mental disorders
- Body pain and difficulty with physical functioning
- Cancer

By using the concept of Reclaim Your Health, I have overcome the effects of being overweight or obese and avoided death, albeit only just; plus, I have been able to reverse the following conditions:

- High blood pressure (Hypertension)
- High LDL cholesterol, low HDL cholesterol, or high levels of triglycerides (Dyslipidemia)
- Type-2 diabetes
- Kidney disease
- Low quality of life
- Mental illnesses such as clinical depression, anxiety, and other mental disorders

Besides the medical conditions that can cause weight gain, sugar is the single most outrageous contributor to obesity. As such, it is crucial to acknowledge the existence of sugar in all forms of plant life.

Researchers reviewed forty-one species of plants and found that, though most plants have 18% to 21% sugar concentrations, the optimal sugar concentration is a bit higher at 23.5%. At the other end of the spectrum, maple syrup, a distillation of the watery maple sap, is quite dense, with a sugar concentration of 65%.

Plants have generally evolved towards the optimum, with several unusually sweet crop plants, such as corn, 40% sugar and potato, 50% sugar.

Three Elements of Sugar

Carbon, oxygen and hydrogen are the common sugar elements in almost all food. Sugar is created by photosynthesis, which uses sunlight to create an energy source essential to the plant and the humans who consume the plants. They convert water and carbon dioxide into carbohydrates (sugar), manufacturing sugar out of thin air.

Plant sugars become cellulose and are synthesised into lignin, the polymer that forms the hard trunks of trees and wood, which have been essential building materials for generations.

Humans and animals need sugar (carbohydrates) as an energy source to fuel their bodies. Still, humans have developed a propensity for consuming more carbohydrates than are required, relevant to an increasing state of sedentariness.

So, our systems have adjusted by storing the excess carbohydrates as fat for later requirements.

Carbohydrates are integral for protein tissue synthesis and are stored in our muscles to govern energy production, speed, concentration, stamina, and fluid balance.

Simple sugars are monosaccharides, including glucose (dextrose), fructose, and galactose. The sugar most commonly used as table sugar is sucrose. This sugar is a disaccharide broken down in the body into fructose and glucose for energy.

There is very little difference between the types of sugar you find in the supermarket (e.g., white, brown, raw, etc.). They are different because of the various processing techniques used in their manufacture.

Consumption, or as some would put it, addiction to sugar, adds excess kilojoules to our diet and contributes significantly to weight gain. Being overweight or obese increases the risk of chronic health problems like high blood pressure, type-2 diabetes and heart disease.

Sugar provides the same amount of energy or kilojoules (kJ) per gram as other digestible carbohydrates such as starch in bread, rice and pasta. However, the World Health Organisation (WHO) recommends that "free" sugars make up no more than 10% of daily kilojoule intake to prevent unhealthy weight gain and dental decay.

Starches

Starch is the most common carbohydrate in the human diet and contains many staple foods. They are widely used in bread, pancakes, cereals, noodles, pasta, porridge, and tortillas. The significant sources of starch intake worldwide are cereals (rice, wheat, and maize) and root vegetables (potatoes and cassava).

Digestive enzymes have problems digesting crystalline structures. Raw starch is digested poorly in the duodenum and small intestine, while bacterial degradation occurs mainly in the colon. When starch is cooked, digestibility is increased.

Before the advent of processed foods, people consumed large amounts of uncooked and unprocessed starch in plants. Microbes within the large intestine ferment the starch, producing short-chain fatty acids, which are used as energy and support the maintenance and growth of the microbes.

More highly processed foods are easily digested and release more glucose in the small intestine, while less starch reaches the large intestine, and the body absorbs more energy.

Starch can be classified as rapidly digestible, slowly digestible and resistant starch. Raw starch granules resist digestion by human enzymes and do not break down into glucose in the small intestine—they reach the large intestine and function as prebiotic dietary fibre.

Fibre

Dietary fibre is found mainly in fruits, vegetables, whole grains, and legumes and is best known for preventing or relieving constipation. Foods containing fibre can provide other health benefits, such as helping maintain a healthy weight and lowering your risk of diabetes, heart disease and cancer.

Whole carbs or simple carbs refer to unprocessed carbohydrates containing fibre found naturally in food; think fruits, legumes, potatoes, and whole grains.

Refined carbs, alternatively known as complex carbs, are stripped of fibre.

Proteins are often referred to as the building blocks of tissue. They are composed of amino acids and break down to form muscle mass and metabolic regulation.

Some great protein sources include natural peanut butter, eggs, quinoa, edamame, plain Greek yoghurt, black beans, and sunflower seeds.

Dietary Fats provide our bodies with energy and support cell growth. There are four main classifications of fats in the food we eat.

Saturated Fats

Saturated fats can cause problems with cholesterol levels, increasing your risk of heart disease. Saturated fats are found in animal-based foods like beef, pork, poultry, full-fat dairy products, eggs, and tropical oils like coconut and palm. Because they are typically solid at room temperature and sometimes called "solid fats".

Unsaturated Fats

They are best described as "good fats" and are preferred by most health professionals, but they are needed as most things are consumed in moderation.

Unsaturated fats are found in meats, lard, and dairy products; trans fats are found in packaged baked goods, potato chips and fast food; Monosaturated fats are found most conveniently in nuts and seeds; and Polyunsaturated fats, an abundance of which are found in fish, seed oils and oysters.

Monounsaturated Fats

Monounsaturated fatty acids, or MUFAs, are a type of unsaturated fat. "Mono", meaning one, signifies that monounsaturated fats have only one double bond and can be found in olive, peanut, and canola oils, avocados, nuts such as almonds, hazelnuts, and pecans and seeds such as pumpkin and sesame seeds.

Polyunsaturated Fats

Polyunsaturated fats are liquid at room temperature and can be found in sunflower, corn, soybean, flaxseed oils, walnuts, fish, and canola oil.

The Importance of Reading Food Labels

Reading food labels is one of the best ways to monitor your added sugar intake. Look for the following names for added sugar and try to avoid either or cut back on the amount or frequency of the foods where they are found:

- brown sugar
- corn sweetener
- corn syrup
- fruit juice concentrates
- high-fructose corn syrup
- honey
- invert sugar
- malt sugar
- molasses
- syrup sugar molecules ending in "ose" (dextrose, fructose, glucose, lactose, maltose, sucrose)

Total sugar, which includes added sugar, is often listed in grams. Note the grams of sugar per serving and the total number of servings. It might only say 5 grams of sugar per serving, but if the expected amount is three or four servings, you can easily consume 20 grams.

Also, keep track of the sugar you add to your food or beverages. About half of the added sugar comes from beverages, including coffee and tea. In May 2017, a study found that nearly two-thirds of coffee and one-third of tea drinkers put sugar or sugary flavourings in their drinks. The researchers also noted that more than 60% of the calories in their beverages came from added sugar.

The Australia New Zealand Food Standards Code (the Code) includes requirements for food labels to have the total amount of sugars in the nutrition information panel.

Total sugars include sugar naturally present in the food and added as an ingredient.

The Code contains requirements for foods that make claims about sugar.

- For example, foods that claim to be "low sugar" cannot contain more than 2.5g of sugar per 100 mL of liquid or 5g per 100g of solid food.

There are also requirements for claims such as "reduced sugar", "x% sugar-free", "no added sugar" and "unsweetened".

Nutrition Information Panels

Various state and federal laws now require nutrition information labels to be printed on all packaged foods, and they must include the average kilojoules for the following items:

- protein
- fat
- saturated fat
- carbohydrate
- sugars
- sodium—a component of salt.

An NIP will include information about other nutrients if a claim is made. For example, if a food has a good source of fibre claim, then the amount of dietary fibre must be shown in the NIP. The NIP must be presented in a standard format showing the average quantity per serving per 100g or 100 mL of a liquid.

There are a few foods that don't require a NIP, for example:

- foods sold unpackaged
- foods made and packaged at the point of sale, such as bread made and sold in a bakery
- herbs, spices, packaged water, tea and coffee because they have no significant nutritional value.

However, a Nutritional Information Panel must be provided if a claim requires nutrition information (for example, a good source of calcium and low fat).

Summary

According to <u>Statista</u>, the number of people who were overweight or obese in 2016 indicates a global health crisis, and it's only getting worse. The following is just a tiny sample of our worldwide problem.

Australia	67.2%
Canada	67.5%
New Zealand	68.0%
USA	70.2%

We have become global consumers of fast food and foods of convenience who have stopped growing our produce and are looking to squeeze meal times into a busy schedule.

Surprise, surprise! Not everything you eat is good for you; even when it tastes so good, you feel it's OK to have another or a little top-up or sneak one while no one is looking.

Processed food is processed to taste good. Why? So you will purchase it again. Make no mistakes: food manufacturers are all about selling you more, a lot more, and a lot more often; that's their game: sell more and make more profit.

Food is fuel; good food can nourish your body, give you energy, and help you live a healthy, meaningful, vitality-filled life. Sure, processed foods with lots of carbohydrates will give you more energy, but ask yourself what happens if the unused carbohydrates (sugar) remain in your system.

Your body stores it for another day or perhaps the day after, or who knows, you may end up locked in a concentration camp without food for months, and all the stored energy will come in handy.

So that delicious little treat you have every night or while no one is watching was manufactured with high sugar levels to be irresistible. The company that made it did so, knowing that 60% of the population is overweight and 10% suffer from diabetes, facts they don't care about because they don't flow through to the bottom line.

Eating more sugar than your liver and muscles can store as glycogen will convert the excess into fat.

When the glucose from your diet does not meet the energy needs of your cells—during fasting or exercise—for example, your body can quickly break down glycogen to produce glucose. If your sugar consumption exceeds your body's immediate energy needs, glucose converts to glycogen and is stored in your liver and muscles. Once these organs can store glycogen, excess glucose converts to fatty acids and triglycerides in your adipose tissue. Similarly, triglycerides break into fatty acids to acetyl-CoA, which enters your mitochondria, fuelling the engine.

After eating, your intestines break down carbohydrates from food into glucose, a type of sugar that goes into your bloodstream, which increases your blood sugar levels.

Your pancreas is an organ that sits just behind your stomach, its job is to release insulin that controls the glucose level in your blood.

Your body makes insulin in a feedback loop based on your blood sugar level and adjusts to changes, similar to your home's air conditioning system releasing cool or warm air as the temperatures rise or fall.

High blood sugar stimulates clusters of special cells, called beta cells, in your pancreas to release insulin. The more glucose you have in your blood, the more insulin your pancreas releases.

Insulin's job is to move glucose into cells for energy while your body stores sugar surplus to your energy requirement in your liver, muscles, and fat cells.

Diabetes *is a chronic health condition that affects how your body turns sugar into energy.* When your blood sugar increases, it signals your pancreas to release insulin.

There are two types of diabetes: *type-1 diabetes is a genetic disorder that often shows up early in life, and type-2 is mainly diet-related and develops over time.* If you have type-1 diabetes, your immune system is attacking and destroying the insulin-producing cells in your pancreas. In contrast, type-2 diabetes can be treated by changing the lifestyle and eating habits of the patient.

Diabetic neuropathy is a type of nerve damage if you have diabetes. Diabetic neuropathy most often damages nerves in your legs and feet. High blood sugar (glucose) can injure nerves throughout your body.

Diabetic neuropathy is a serious diabetes complication that may affect as many as 50% of people with diabetes. Some people have mild symptoms, while others can be painful and disabling. Excessive sugar levels in your system can cause diabetic neuropathy, with symptoms ranging from pain and numbness in your legs and feet to problems with your digestive system, urinary tract, blood vessels and heart.

I should know because the peripheral neuropathy caused by my type-2 diabetes delivered levels of nerve pain that could only be relieved with high doses of Lyrica.

Lyrica is a controlled substance. It's classified as a Schedule V prescription drug. Schedule V drugs have accepted medical uses, but they also have the potential to cause psychological or physical dependence, and as a result, the drug could be misused. While this medication brought relief from the icepick and burn pain, I felt in my feet and legs the drug has an extensive list of side effects that sometimes offset the drug's ability to act as a central nerve blocker, reducing pain.

Lyrica may cause dizziness, drowsiness, oedema (fluid retention), particularly in the feet or hands, weight gain, angioedema (swelling of the face, mouth, or neck), headache, tremors, abnormal thinking, dry mouth, constipation, blurred vision, lack of energy, and potential changes in some laboratory test results such as creatine kinase, and ECG changes.

As a person who for twenty years has suffered from kidney issues, Lyrica was a drug I needed to reduce, but unfortunately, not one you can stop taking quickly without serious side effects.

"Your life changes the moment you make a new, congruent, and committed decision."

– Anthony Robbins

Chapter 5
My Why

Recently, I have been reminded why I decided to write this book and recorded hundreds of one-minute messages that I posted on Instagram. The answer is best summarised by telling you my WHY, not why I have done these things, although the two are closely linked for obvious reasons, but my WHY, my passion, and my desire to make a difference in someone else life.

My WHY is simple, "Health is a Choice", but it's a choice most of us never make because our health is something we take for granted.

I want to reach out to as many people as possible and tell them, show them, and be an example to them that no matter your age, underlying health conditions or regrets, you can change your lifestyle habits and reinvent your health.

To understand the importance of defining your "WHY", you must first understand the concept.

While I don't profess to be an expert in this space, I have read several books on the subject and spent several hours delving into the complexities of digging deep into my psyche while reflecting on the history that brought me to this space.

In his books *Find Your Why* and *Start With Why*, Simon Sinek tells many stories about business people who have mastered the art of turning their WHY into a company culture that helped drive that business to achieve outstanding results.

Specifically, Simon refers to Apple Inc. and Southwest Airlines as companies with powerful WHYs that are very clear and compelling. He further explains how they have worked to develop the crucial concept of the Golden Circle.

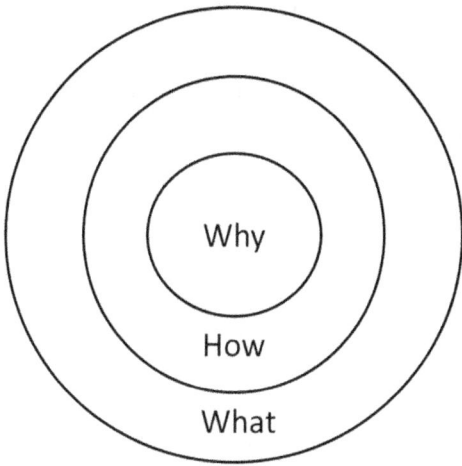

WHAT's are the products, services and job functions we perform?

HOWs are values, guiding principles and actions that make us stand out.

The WHY defines what the individual or organisation stands for, and it's the collective purpose, cause or belief.

Most of us think about the Golden Circle by communicating outside in (WHAT-HOW-WHY). Those with the capacity to inspire do it differently. They think, act and speak from the inside out (WHY-HOW-WHAT).

Every one of us has a WHY, a deep-seated purpose, cause or belief that is the source of our passion and inspiration and is part of the fulfilment we seek.

The difference between happiness and fulfilment is between liking and loving something, and I believe fulfilment comes when our job connects directly to our WHY.

- Happiness comes from what we do.
- Fulfilment comes from why we do it.

Apple INC and Southeast Airlines have achieved outstanding growth in both businesses. Their WHY has changed the culture of the companies.

While culture is not essential for me in articulating the importance of what I was doing on Instagram and Twitter, this book may provide many a better understanding of the passion that drives me daily.

I spent many hours creating one paragraph that encapsulates the passion and emotion that has driven me to write this book and devote so much time trying to convince people that "Health is a Choice" and choices have consequences.

I failed to be the husband and father I could be when I failed to fight for my health and the quality of my life.

My WHY

I want my wife and three daughters to see me as an inspiration to them and others by demonstrating that adversity can be overcome and, regardless of a person's age, health can be dramatically improved by changing the habits of a lifetime.

As for my HOW and WHAT, perhaps another time.

Compare the two photographs below and judge for yourself.

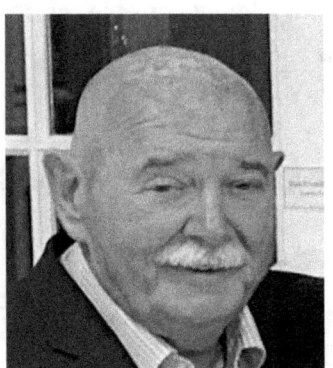 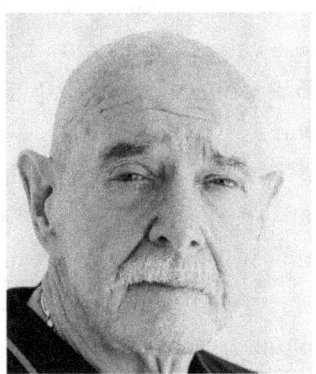

September 2020   February 2023

Chapter 6
After the Dash

Knowledge and Wisdom

The accumulation of knowledge is often associated with a person's intelligence, yet in the absence of wisdom relevant to that knowledge, said knowledge has limited or no value.

Knowledge of my various health issues and what caused them were almost always delivered by doctors who advised of the need to accept that there was little or nothing that could be done to reverse or fix my medical issues.

I did not know at these vital moments in my health journey that if I were able to change my lifestyle habits, I would have improved the quality of my life, extended the length of my life and improved the quality of my life.

Headstones contain the date of birth and death of the person buried, separated by the "-". I had no say in my birth date, but I have a say in the date chiselled in stone on the other side of my "-".

I have no idea what date I will die, nor do I want to know, and what I do every day with my exercise and diet is purely designed to push the date of my death backwards and improve the quality of my life. I have and will continue to fight daily to reverse the medical conditions that have stolen the quality of my life and fractured my relationship with my wife and children.

While I have come to cherish my life, I don't understand why others do things every day that put their lives at risk, some as part of their profession, others who push the limits and thrive on the thrill associated with that danger.

Our health influences the date on the other side of everyone's "-" yet health is something we all take for granted until something changes our perspective. Knowledge supported by a doctor's wisdom and a desire to change the habits of a lifetime can and will change everything related to our health and the quality of the life we choose to live.

This week has seen day surgery for an endoscopic and colonoscopy examination and reasonably large polyp removal.

While waiting for the biopsy results, I do what most of us do: I use Doctor Google to search all the unpronounceable words in the doctor's initial examination report.

There is also a significant growth on my chest, which I have been waiting to see my dermatologist. Having had several skin cancers surgically removed and what must be hundreds frozen, I have become somewhat knowledgeable on the subject.

My scorecard is one small melanoma, several cycle cell carcinomas, and four Squamous Cell Carcinomas. Still, the latest Squamous Cell Carcinoma is much larger than anything previously detected, is located between my peck muscles, and is very advanced. So, surgery is booked just before Christmas, and I will be back to get the results of my gastroenterologist in the same week. It could be a great Christmas present or set the scene for a reasonably shitty one.

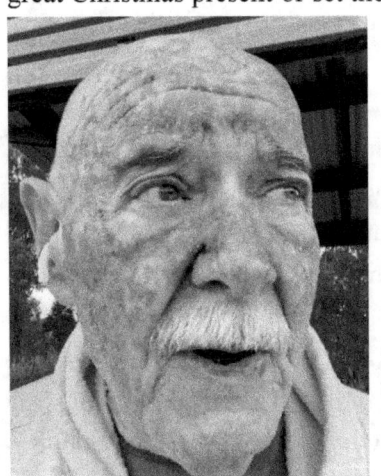

Following this, I needed to remove a small section of my left ear. The biopsy returned with a poor result, requiring further surgery and chemotherapy. As you can see from the image, skin cancer damage over my face was extensive. The treatment left me feeling like a snake shedding its skin while open sores were all over my face, which then became infected and required antibiotics to help fight the infection.

Considering that these issues did not just suddenly arise, they had been brewing for a long time before either condition became urgent enough to warrant seeing my doctor. The cancer on my chest looked like most of the other skin cancers I have had, but it has doubled in size over a few weeks and changed consistency, which is a sign that this is a more significant issue than I thought.

Several weeks after the polyps had been removed, I was advised they were pre-cancerous (pre-cancerous colon polyps, if left untreated, can progress into colon cancer). In contrast, the skin cancer on my chest was removed. At that same time, my dermatologist advised I had two small but deep Scuarmous cancers on my right cheek that needed to be removed by a plastic surgeon.

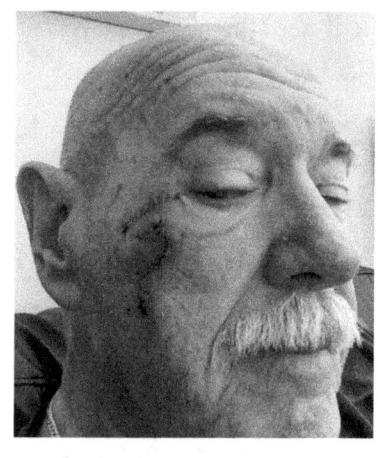

The plastic surgery removed the cancer, and the pathology confirmed it was a Scuarmous cell carcinoma that had reached my cheekbone but had not penetrated the bone.

When I reflect on my medical history, the one thing common to all of my medical conditions is that I did nothing to prevent these medical events from happening.

Ignorance is not an excuse; stupidity on reflection is a good description of my response and actions. I don't believe I am the only person who feels good medical advice will get you through your medical crisis. I had no idea any medical conditions would happen, but if I trace them back to their root cause, I was overweight and had been for most of my life. I was happy with my identity and weight; I didn't know better.

Knowledge is defined as "what is learned", while wisdom "applies that knowledge in such a way as to achieve the desired outcome".

Had I known that my eating habits would damage my kidneys, liver, and heart, elevate my blood pressure, give me type 2 diabetes, cause a stroke, become clinically depressed, and attempt suicide, would I have kept doing what I was doing?

So, the absence of knowledge about the issues my lifestyle habits would cause left me unable to make the required corrections to my lifestyle habits.

At this point, you may wonder whether you need to take stock of your medical situation and change some of your lifestyle habits. If so, then do the following.

- Weigh yourself naked
- Measure your height
- Measure your waist circumference
- Measure your hip circumference
- Measure your chest circumference
- Calculate your BMI

Go online to calculate your BMI, and if you don't like the answer, what will you do about it?

As a guide, I have listed below the BMI scale to see where your eating and exercise habits, assisted by your lifestyle, have placed you on the scale.

Below 18.5	Underweight
18.5—24.9	Healthy
25.0—29.9	Overweight
30.0 and Above	Obese

The effects of Being Overweight or Obese are significant. If you think you are overweight or your BMI is higher than 30.0, you are obese, and you risk developing serious complications that will either shorten your life or reduce the quality of your life.

I know because I lived in denial most of my life. The consequences of that denial have caused me considerable difficulties and more continuous pain than most people would be capable of bearing. Add to that the pain and hardship I have caused my wife and daughters, and you should have a compelling argument for why you need to make changes.

Listed below AGAIN are the health conditions that can occur due to being overweight. The items shown in red are conditions I have and am currently being treated for.

- High blood pressure (Hypertension)
- High LDL cholesterol, low HDL cholesterol, or high levels of triglycerides (Dyslipidemia)
- Type-1 and 2 diabetes
- Coronary heart disease
- Stroke
- Gallbladder disease
- Osteoarthritis (a breakdown of cartilage and bone within a joint)
- Sleep apnoea and breathing problems
- Low quality of life
- Mental illnesses such as clinical depression, anxiety, and other mental disorders
- Body pain and difficulty with physical functioning

Accept Your Fate

OK, assuming you have taken your measurements and been online to determine your BMI and have considered the consequences of your continued denial that you have a weight problem, what will you do about it?

Accept your fate and wait until you experience a medical incident, and hope someone close to you understands what needs to happen and takes the necessary action. Well, it's unlikely someone will be around, and even if they are, what are the chances they will have the training or knowledge needed to care for you while waiting for an ambulance or medical assistance?

I have always been under the care of an MD and several specialists who knew how to treat my medical conditions, and the intervention of these professionals, the care and the medications they prescribed were critical to my recovery and are the sole reason I have survived these crises recover my health and have been able to write this book.

I can't say the same for four friends and loved ones in the last twelve months.

John (not his real name) suffered a heart attack in his front yard and survived, thanks to the quick and decisive intervention of a neighbour who applied CPR for over thirty minutes until an ambulance arrived.

Paul (not his real name) fainted in his backyard and was rushed to the hospital, where the doctors decided they needed to perform open-heart surgery. While on the operating table, Paul experienced a bilateral stroke that affected both sides of his brain; after consulting with his wife, the doctors turned the life support system off, and Paul passed within minutes.

Frank (not his real name) experienced a stroke that affected the left side of his brain, and while he recovered, the use of his arm and leg he now talks with a noticeable difference from how he spoke previously.

Judy, my mother-in-law, suffered a stroke while on a tour of NSW country and was transported to Mildura Hospital in Victoria. After several weeks of care, we arranged for the Flying Doctor Service to fly her back to Sydney, where she was admitted to a hospital near our home. While at this hospital, it was discovered she had metastasised cancer and passed within six months of the stroke.

These four people and their health issues confirmed why I needed to intensify my effort to lose the weight that dictated my health and the quality of my life for many years.

Since September 2020, we have spent a lot of time in the mornings walking and talking with Jacqui, and when she needed to get home and get ready for work, I would keep walking. I used this time to listen to various audio and podcasts to help me reconfirm what I was doing and why I needed to focus on improving my health.

Significantly, these audios were not about weight loss, exercise, or health; rather, they carried a message that reaffirmed the importance of my belief in myself and my self-esteem. Over time, these audio and audiobooks affirmed my passion for wanting others to understand that it is possible for anyone, regardless of their age or health, to improve the quality of their life and learn to live a meaningful life while reclaiming their health.

My passion for sharing my health journey became more potent, and that's when I decided to start recording sixty-second snippets and publishing them on Instagram.

Jacqui and I walk together daily, and during one of these walks, she told me how she has dealt with my thirty years of medical history. She spoke about two words, fear and anger, so I asked if she would be prepared to record these feelings for me to post on Instagram. This recording confirmed why this health journey has been so crucial for me. I wanted other people like me who live in denial to understand how their families might feel about them being overweight or in poor health. And many other people got the message based on the high response and comments.

Jacqui's anger stemmed from the belief that I didn't care enough about my health to do something about it, and this neglect implied that I did not love her or our children enough, while her fear was centred around what life was going to be like without me.

Jacqui lost her mother and father in the last seven years, and while grief is very personal, sharing the journey with her has allowed me to see how poorly she has coped with that loss and understand how my death would be soul-destroying.

On a separate occasion, Jacqui told me about a conversation with one of our daughters where Jacqui was asked to interpret a dream. My daughter described an accident where all five of us were on a train that collided with a car at a crossing. The train derailed and flipped on its side, and Jacqui managed to get our three daughters to safety, but I was trapped under a seat, and Jacqui was unable to free me. The train was on fire and Jacqui had to leave me and ensure our three daughters were safe.

My daughter wanted to know the answer to one question: if daddy were still alive, you wouldn't leave him there, would you?

Until I committed to writing this book, I had no idea what damage I had done to my three beautiful daughters. Fearful of the outcome of my health drove one of my daughters to nightmares about me and my safety and her concern that Jacqui may decide to leave me behind to save our children.

The people you love and those who love you care about you and want nothing but the best for you in all aspects of your life, but rarely, if ever, will they tell you what they are feeling. Their fear and anger will never be fully known because most people shy away from the hard conversations about weight and health. After all, they don't know how to broach the subject.

In some of my posts on Instagram, I have told the story of being in the ICU attached to all sorts of devices, and when I opened my eyes to see Jacqui and our three beautiful daughters standing at my bed, their eyes filled with tears. If I could leave just one impression in the minds of the people who read this book or have listened to my sixty-second post on Instagram, it would be this very picture.

Please close your eyes, see yourself in that ICU bed, and replace my family with yours.

I want you to flip the vision and find yourself standing at the foot of the bed, looking at your wife or one of your children.

What would you do, what would you give, what would you say, what would you change for that person in the ICU bed to live an entirely natural and healthy life?

Extend Your Life

Every person of sound mind would want to extend their life; however, wanting and doing are two different things, given none of us knows what health issues are just waiting to surface. But what if you knew a health issue would strike you down five years from now, and what could you do to prevent it from happening? Would you commit to making the required changes?

The answer is, of course, you would; who in their right mind would not do whatever it took to extend their life?

The trouble is you don't know what medical issue will strike you down, so the best way to describe this is to outline an example you can easily understand.

All the people who have replaced tyres on their cars will understand this example.

After the tyres have been fitted, balanced, and inflated, the car should have a wheel alignment to ensure maximum mileage from your new tyres.

What do you think happens to new tyres when?

- The car hits a large pothole.
- Nail/screw puncture
- Under-inflated tyres
- Over-inflated tyres
- Sharp objects
- Leaking valve
- Ripped tyre
- Damaged rim
- Blowout

The loss of tyre pressure caused by all of the above is not always apparent, and we keep driving until it becomes noticeable or the damage to the tyre and rim brings the vehicle to a halt. Drive a car with under or over-inflated tyre pressure, and the tyre wears unevenly and needs to be replaced.

The same is true with your health, given that most of us have an unknown health issue slowly developing and waiting for the most inconvenient time to surface. With a lack of knowledge, ignorance or, worst still, denial of any symptoms that are stealing the quality of your health as slowly as the air leaks from a damaged tyre, you inevitably will be faced with one of the following issues:

Hit a Large Pothole—**Stroke, Aneurysm**
Nail/Screw Puncture—**Stroke, Heart Attack**
Under-inflated Tyres—**Nausea, Fatigue**
Over-Inflated Tyres—**Enlarged Heart, Replacement**
Sharp Objects—**Stitches**
Leaking Valve—**Heart Valve Replacement**
Ripped Tyre—**Bypass Surgery**

Damaged Rim—**Stroke**

Blowout—**Heart Attack**

Damaged tyres are identified during inspection or when the loss of air pressure in the tyre becomes so noticeable.

Health issues are no different to the pressure in your tyres; once identified and after examination by your doctor and confirmed by medical tests, it requires either repair or intervention.

You can either wait until your health (tyre pressure) declines and your doctor orders a test that identifies an issue that needs to be surgically corrected or prescribes medication to mask the condition. Alternatively, you can start slowly changing the habits that deflate your health.

The Choice is Yours

The choice has always been yours, but if you are anything like me, you will avoid changing your habits because it all seems too hard. However, you need to understand that your failure to make that decision now has consequences that aren't nice and that regrets will do nothing for you other than make you miserable.

Regrets come from "I wonder what would be different in my life if only I had ***".

Failure to change your habits will affect you and all the people you love and who love you.

I had an appointment recently with my dermatologist to remove a Squamous Cell Carcinoma, and I had not told my daughters why I was visiting the doctor. I did not mention it because I believed they had heard enough about my medical conditions and were concerned about causing them unnecessary duress.

My youngest daughter, who is in her final year of dentistry, found out about Squamous Cell Carcinoma and, given this cancer is part of her study, had a great deal of knowledge about this cancer. Paige was upset with me for not telling her and her sisters and expressed similar concerns to my wife, Jacqui.

Fear and anger were the primary feelings she spoke to me about, and again, I seemed to trivialise the issue and did not think about them enough to share what was happening.

From my perspective, I trivialise my medical issues as part of my coping mechanism. I stopped sharing these issues with the family because I had burdened them enough.

Sometimes, our choices are selfish, and we make them for the wrong reasons, trying to protect our loved ones from unnecessary worry. My philosophy has always been, "It isn't a problem until it is confirmed as a problem", so I will deal with it when I know its extent.

When it comes to your health, the point I need to impress upon you is simple: if you think you are OK, then you're not; if you know you're OK, that knowledge must have been created from an authoritative source, a second, a professional opinion.

- In my twenties, I thought I was indestructible.
- In my thirties, I carried a little extra weight and thought that wasn't a problem.
- In my forties, I was still carrying that weight, and I was in denial that my health had declined.
- In my fifties, I was dealing with the consequences of that denial.
- In my sixties, I was struggling to stay alive.
- The lights came on in my seventies, and I decided to reclaim my health.

The choice is yours; you can pretend you don't have a health issue or you are not overweight or unhealthy. Statistics don't lie. Instead, these statistics paint a very sobering picture of our world and the number of people who are overweight and obese. Alarmingly, that number is growing at an alarming annual rate.

According to WHO, worldwide obesity has nearly tripled since 1975.

- In 2016, over 1.9 billion adults eighteen years and older were overweight. Of these, over 650 million were obese.
- 39% of adults aged eighteen years and over were overweight in 2016, and 13% were obese.
- Most of the world's population lives in countries where overweight and obese kill more people than underweight.
- 39 million children under the age of five were overweight or obese in 2020

- Over 340 million children and adolescents aged five to nineteen were overweight or obese in 2016

Obesity is preventable.

If Health is a Choice, why would we not choose good health and a life filled with all we could ever want? The answer is simple: we don't think about our health like that. We don't think about it at all, that is until something happens that draws our attention to that health issue.

Every day, we think about work, finances, love, sex, what we will have for dinner or lunch and a thousand other thoughts, but the essential thing that makes everything we do in our life possible is that we take for granted and treat as irrelevant; we assume is not a problem is our health. Until we hit a speed bump in the middle of our life's highway, we never saw coming.

If you have a regular checkup with your doctor, they will probably run a series of blood tests to determine any underlying issues that may need to be addressed. On the other hand, if you don't see a doctor regularly, I strongly recommend you find one you are comfortable with and put regular medical checkups in place.

Your doctor will probably run the following test as part of any regular checkup.

Tests for Heart
Blood tests

- Electrocardiogram (ECG)
- Exercise stress test

Test for Kidney
Blood Test

- Serum Creatinine
- Glomerular Filtration Rate(GFR)
- Blood Urea Nitrogen (BUN)

Urine Test

- Urinalysis
- Albumin-to-Creatinine Ratio (ACR)
- Creatinine Clearance

Test for Liver
Blood Test

- alanine transaminase (ALT)
- aspartate aminotransferase (AST)
- alkaline phosphatase (ALP)
- albumin
- bilirubin

The good news. All you have to do is ask your doctor to run these urine and blood tests for you and then review the results with them. These tests should be part of the standard treatment of care you are receiving from our doctor, and if they have not run these tests for you, either request they do or find a doctor who will run them for you and do it annually.

Summary

My personality type is Choleric. "Someone with a choleric personality is typically *extroverted, goal-oriented, and ambitious*. As a result, many are natural-born leaders. However, they can also be short-tempered and even violent due to their personality." So, understanding how I think and approach problems should give insight into why this subject has become an extremely passionate journey.

I am angry with myself for allowing my health to be slowly sucked away, and in my haste to live my life, I have come close to losing it, but it doesn't need to be that way for you as long as you create action steps from this book that help you take the actions required to Reclaim Your Health.

If you still have doubts, find the best nursing home in your area and ask them for a guided tour. Please have a good hard look at the residents sitting in their rooms staring out the window, sitting in visitor rooms, being entertained with mindless games to help wield away the hours. Visit the dining rooms and ask yourself if you want to join them for dinner every night.

My mother-in-law was admitted to one of the best aged care facilities in Sydney after a stroke that took the use of the left side of her body. I watched her being hoisted onto the toilets or into the shower by underpaid staff who were too few because these aged care facilities couldn't find all the needed staff.

Regarding the quality of life, I do not regard this as anything I would ever wish to endure while committing several hundred thousand dollars to upfront and weekly support fees.

"But like they say, it's not the years in your life that count; it's the life in your years. And I sure as hell was going to make my life count."

– Jay McLean

Chapter 7
Reclaim Your Health

Fatalists believe we cannot change our destiny, that the day we were born and the day we will die are already determined. Whatever we do to change our future is always part of our future, and nothing I can do, including stepping in front of a bus, is anything other than fulfilling my destiny.

These same people would have you believe that my health journey has been nothing but a journey and that I would always be a borderline casualty of some medical condition but survive. This journey and this book occurred because they would always be part of my life, and what I did to improve my health, what I recorded as part of my daily journal, and what I posted on social media would influence some, but not others.

For this to be true, nothing I could do or say would ever influence anyone other than those whom fate intended to change.

On the other side of this argument is my belief that I can influence the date of my death through my actions and decisions. By suffering and surviving these medical conditions, the lessons I have learned and applied and the activities I have committed to do daily will affect the length and quality of my life.

Retrain Your Mind

My father left his marriage and two children when I was twelve years old and moved to a different state, so I lost the regular contact a boy needs with the one person in his life that prepares them to be the man they need to become. However, he left me with one comment that rattled around in my head and still impacts me whenever I allow it out of the dark closet, which is my subconscious.

"He will never amount to anything."

The psychological damage from this one comment passed by my father limited my ability to believe in myself and reach my true potential until I learnt how to overcome this damage. The thoughts that ran through my head diminished my ability to make positive changes in my life and foster confidence in myself.

Negative self-talk can be stressful and limit your success until you find a way to overcome the issue.

We tend to:

- Remember traumatic experiences better than positive ones.
- Recall insults better than praise.
- React more strongly to negative stimuli.
- Think about negative things more frequently than positive ones.
- Respond more strongly to adverse events than to equally positive ones.

For example, you might be having a great day at work when an offhand comment that you find irritating, and you are stewing over those words for the rest of the day and revisiting them repeatedly.

When you get home from work, and someone asks you how your day was, you reply that it was terrible—even though it was overall quite good despite that one negative incident.

Below are a few suggestions that may help you overcome your negative subconscious and throw away comments from a father justifying why he no longer wants to be part of your family. While the statement still lives in my mind, and these techniques have helped me lessen their impact on my belief system, I am still dealing with them.

- Mind dump negative thoughts before you go to bed
- Change your environment to improve your thinking
- Reduce TV time and replace it with books
- Take a digital detox once a month
- Listen to more audiobooks and podcasts to gain knowledge
- Spend time amongst positive, helpful people
- Use meditation when negative thoughts happen
-

Footnote:

During one of the few times my father and I spent together, as he watched me playing with my three daughters on our lounge room floor, I believe seeing me as a loving father caring for his children, he was filled with regret; regret what he could have had but chose to walk away.

While my father's comment, "He will never amount to anything", had a negative impact on my belief system for many years and still to this day comes front of my mind when things aren't going exactly the way I want, I believe what he said was out of spite and directed more towards my mother than reflecting his feelings about me.

I have learnt to use comments like my father's and negative comments from other people I have associated with as a catalyst for change. We don't have to accept criticisms or comments as gospel but as input to refocus our self-belief systems and use them as turning points to refocus our efforts.

If my father had meant what he said, my success, achievements, and recognition would have caused him to know I was not the failure he had predicted.

While our body needs food for energy and water for hydration to function properly, our brain needs stimulation and positive input to cope with the complexity of today's lifestyle. The human body can survive three to five days without water and go days or weeks without food. Still, our brains need to be stimulated, focused, and filled with positive thoughts and knowledge to sustain our lifestyles and improve the quality of our lives.

We are bombarded with information delivered by radio, visual, auditory (movies), television, internet, social media, and printed material, including books, newspapers, and blogs. Deciding on the source of this information we allow into our heads should be predicated on the accuracy of that information and nothing else. Some are accurate, some are questionable, and some are rubbish.

I heard it said this week that "a person who does not read the newspaper, listen to the radio, watch the news and current affairs programs or use social media in any form is better educated than someone who uses all of them". The point being made is simple: we have stopped reporting the news. Instead, we are manufacturing the way news is presented. Donald Trump called it fake news, but it has become a reporter or a media owner's perspective, and it is being used to persuade us to change our thinking.

Our brains process and retain information differently based on the delivery mechanism. Reading involves several brain functions, including visual and auditory processes, phonemic awareness, fluency, comprehension, etc. Reading gives the brain more time to stop, think, process, and imagine the narrative in front of us, processing what is written, from the letters to the words to the sentences to the stories themselves, boosting brain activity.

It follows that information delivered to us visually via radio, visual, auditory (movies), television and the internet sometimes does not allow time to stop, think, process, and imagine the narrative because they are incorporated into the delivery by the media.

While I have never been an active reader, I am committed to reading leadership, motivation, success, self-help, and management books. I have made this one of my new habits that form part of my identity; I have dedicated time to the process and a space in my home where I read for a minimum of ten minutes or ten pages daily. I also listen to the same book using Audible because I absorb the content more effectively by listening and reading the same material.

I learnt many years ago to use a highlighter pen and sticky tabs to categorise the book by sections relevant and essential to me. This process allowed me to quickly rescan areas of a book that have greater relevance for me and the changes I am trying to make.

I listen to daily motivations from three key motivational speakers, Darren Hardy, John Maxwell, Mel Robbins, and Keith Abraham, plus a thirty-minute health and weight loss education. I dedicate this time to retraining my brain to counter all the negative and subconscious thoughts continually trying to hold me back.

Understanding more about the human body, how it responds to food, and the exercises have allowed me to reclaim my health and overcome several medical conditions that, if left unchecked, would unquestionably shorten my life.

What You Put in Your Stomach

Being born in 1948 placed me in a time zone when the foods I consumed were organically grown and free of synthetic chemicals, pesticides, fertilisers, or genetically modified organisms. While you can still buy organically grown foods today, the cost of these products, in some instances, is 20% higher than non-organically grown food.

Cost aside, studies show that crops as varied as wheat, maize, soybeans, and field peas contain less protein, zinc, and iron when grown under increased carbon dioxide levels. In contrast, many other crops have already suffered losses in these nutrients.

With all these changes in the quality of the food we eat, the healthcare industry suggests we supplement our dietary requirements with vital vitamins and minerals to achieve and maintain good health.

The need for vitamins to be balanced with macronutrients, carbs, and fats is necessary to maintain daily bodily functions, such as cell reproduction and growth, and most importantly, the processing of energy in cells.

Both quality and quantity are of utmost importance for overall health. However, quality may win slightly over quantity in this weight-loss debate, but remember, you can still gain weight if you overeat healthy foods.

Scientists tell us we need to sustain a healthy life. So if we agree on that undeniable fact, the big question is, what can we do about it? How can we ensure our bodies receive all the proper nutrients and vitamins?

The answer is simple: supplement what you eat with vitamins and minerals and ensure your water is purified, not just filtered.

Although most vitamins are derived from plants, they are often consumed indirectly from higher up the food chain in foods of animal origin, including meat, dairy and eggs, sometimes in forms that have already undergone some form of initial tailoring for bioactivity. Alternatively, enzymatic tailoring is to achieve their bioactive forms.

A person who will not invest in themselves does not know a good investment when it's staring back at them in the mirror. Ensure your diet has the correct balance of carbohydrates, fats, and proteins, and ensure your weight remains healthy for your age. Buy organic whenever possible and invest in supplements to support your body.

Let's debate about organic vs non-organic to one side, and let's not even consider the issue associated with the extra cost of purchasing organic foods. Instead, let's agree that the quality of the food and water we eat and drink is declining. Declining quality will only continue and, at the same time, force us to invest in technology to deliver the standard our future well-being requires.

"One should eat to live, not live to eat."

– Moliere

Physical Activity and Exercise

When you exercise, your body releases chemicals such as dopamine and endorphins in your brain that make you happy. Not only is your brain dumping out feel-good chemicals, but exercise also helps your brain eliminate chemicals that make you feel stressed and anxious.

Simple Rule: eat before exercise, and your body will convert what you have eaten into energy. Suppose your physical activity and exercise are designed to help you lose weight. In that case, I recommend walking at least forty-five minutes before breakfast daily, rain, hail or shine, during summer and winter. Walk on an empty stomach; the only energy source available is the fat your body has stored. You will need to get your active minutes above eighty, and if you walk slower than the average person, it's worth noting this may not be counted as active minutes.

Active minutes are calculated through an equivalent metabolic metric, which measures the intensity of a particular physical exercise by comparing it against a base rate. The base rate is roughly an average person's resting metabolic rate, which estimates your body's caloric burn when you sit still. However, going for a leisurely walk requires twice as much energy as you do when you rest.

Measuring the number of steps and active minutes has become easier with the available technologies on smartwatches and phones and the various built-in apps available to help measure and record this activity.

You don't need to engage in physical exercises, like running, gym workouts, and other personal training activities that get your heart rate to its upper limits. Walking has been identified as one of the best exercises anyone can undertake. You need to walk approximately fifteen thousand steps daily and a pace recorded by Fitbit or Apple Watch as over a hundred active minutes.

Walking and running are both aerobic cardiovascular exercises and include the following health benefits:

- helps you lose weight or maintain a healthy weight
- increases stamina
- boosts immune system
- helps prevent or manage chronic conditions
- can extend your life

Just thirty minutes of moderate cardiovascular exercise three times a week reduces anxiety and depression, improving your mood and, possibly, your self-esteem.

Brisk walking is an excellent moderate-intensity exercise for weight loss, reducing health risks and building fitness, and fewer injuries than running.

Physical Fitness

You don't need to be a marathon runner or an elite athlete to derive significant benefits from physical fitness and the activity associated with that achievement.

When you consider the most significant gains come from:

- When an individual goes from being sedentary to becoming moderately active.
- When an individual goes from being moderately active to very active.
- The most significant gains were achieved between the lowest fitness group and the next lowest fitness group.

Healthy adults who are not considered physically fit have a mortality risk of 4.5 times greater than those who are physically fit. Surprisingly, an individual's fitness level was a more important predictor of death than established risk factors such as:

- smoking
- high blood pressure
- high cholesterol
- diabetes

There is mounting evidence in the scientific community that physical activity and physical fitness have a powerful influence on chronic diseases.

- All causes of death (mortality)
- High blood pressure (Hypertension)
- High LDL cholesterol, low HDL cholesterol, or high levels of triglycerides (Dyslipidemia)
- Type-1 and 2 diabetes
- Coronary heart disease
- Stroke
- Gallbladder disease

- Osteoarthritis (a breakdown of cartilage and bone within a joint)
- Sleep apnoea and breathing problems
- Low quality of life
- Mental illnesses such as clinical depression, anxiety, and other mental disorders
- Body pain and difficulty with physical functioning

Cardiovascular Fitness

Cardiovascular fitness is achieved through sustained physical activity. It is measured by a person's ability to deliver oxygen to the working muscles and is affected by heart rate, stroke volume, cardiac output, and maximal oxygen consumption.

Increase your aerobic capacity, your general metabolism rises, muscle metabolism will be enhanced, haemoglobin will grow, buffers in the bloodstream will increase venous return, stroke volume will improve, and the blood bed will adapt readily to the varying demands on your body.

These cardiovascular results will directly affect muscular endurance and impact strength and flexibility.

Summary

This health journey has had its challenges for me. Had I not been in denial for as long as I was, had I not been the fool I was, had I heard the messages that were put to me rather than listened to whatever I wanted to hear, this journey may not have been so challenging.

If health is really a choice, and it was there for me to choose, I can't help but wonder what my life would have looked like had I believed my health could be whatever I wanted it to be.

I believe everything happens for a purpose; my poor health choices have helped shape the lives of Jacqui and my three daughters, and I have to believe in a good way.

Despite whatever I believe, I owe them an apology. I know it hasn't been easy for my family at times, and I also know that hardship has prepared them for something that will happen in life and that they had to endure may never become apparent.

I also believe my purpose brought me to this book, and this book can change just one life; then, all I have endured was worth the price.

Let health be a daily choice for the balance of your life.

"Physical fitness is not only one of the most important keys to a healthy body, it is the basis of dynamic and creative intellectual activity."

– John F. Kennedy

Chapter 8
Soil Degradation

Soil degradation happens when the quality of soil declines and diminishes its capacity to support animal and plant life. Soil can lose specific physical, chemical or biological attributes that underpin the web of life.

Soil erosion is a part of soil degradation when the topsoil and nutrients are lost naturally, such as wind, flood, or human actions, such as poor land management.

First and foremost, I am not a greenie or a tree hugger. However, I believe our health is dictated by the quality of what we put into our bodies. The quality of the plant life and livestock we consume is impacted by the quality of the soil and water used to produce this food.

Unquestionably, the quality of the soil we grow our plant life has degraded over the last hundred years, affecting the quality of the plant life we eat. To counter the degradation of our soil, farmers use fertilisers and other artificial techniques rather than managing the quality of our soil to ensure the soil has a higher nutrient value and is microbe-rich.

The different chemical, physical, and biological properties of soil interact in complex ways, determining its potential and capacity to produce healthy and nutritious crops.

Soil quality can be defined by its compatibility, erosion, and fertility. The term also refers to the soil's structural integrity, preventing erosion and loss of plant nutrients and organic matter. Integrating these properties and the resulting productivity level is called "soil quality".

Soil quality should not be limited to soil productivity but should encompass environmental quality, human and animal health, and food safety and quality. There is inadequate information on how soil quality changes directly affect food quality or indirectly affect human and animal health.

Soil quality and biological properties have received less emphasis than chemical and physical properties because their effects are difficult to measure, predict, or quantify. Increased infiltration, aeration, macropores, aggregate size, aggregate stability, soil organic matter, decreased bulk density, soil resistance, erosion, and nutrient runoff often indicate improved soil quality.

Environmental scientists worldwide agree we are losing the capacity to use our soil effectively enough to produce crops of the same quality as we did a hundred years ago. We are effectively sucking the nutrients out of the ground and using fertilisers with the knowledge that those fertilisers will help growers harvest more productive quantities.

Coupled with the salinity levels of our water tables consistently rising, our ability to harvest plants with nutritional value is essential to humans' growth and development. We have a problem our next generation will inherit and cannot reverse.

Phytonutrients are natural compounds in plant foods such as vegetables, fruits, whole grains, and legumes. These plant compounds benefit from working with other essential nutrients to promote good health. Among the benefits of phytonutrients are antioxidant and anti-inflammatory activities. Phytonutrients may also enhance immunity and intercellular communication, repair DNA damage from exposure to toxins and detoxify carcinogens.

These essential elements of our dietary intake help sustain and restore our health.

We are what we eat and then the protein we eat. The quality of that is dependent on what that animal eats. A well-balanced diet will improve health and overall body composition, but the brain-gut connection can make us feel better, healthier, and more robust. Eating well is a simple strategy that will reduce our risk of chronic disease and improve the condition of our genes. Common-sense recommendations such as low sugar, low salt, and a good variety of nutrients are best to sustain a healthy lifestyle.

Examples of Soil Degradation

Soil degradation is the physical, chemical and biological decline in soil quality. It can be the loss of organic matter, decline in soil fertility, structural condition, erosion, adverse changes in salinity, acidity or alkalinity, and the effects of toxic chemicals, pollutants or excessive flooding. Soil degradation can involve:

- water erosion
- wind erosion
- salinity
- loss of organic matter
- fertility decline
- soil acidity or alkalinity
- structure decline
- mass movement
- soil contamination

Erosion degrades the land, resulting in its inability to support plant life, which converts carbon dioxide into oxygen. Better land management can help keep soils intact and grow more plant life. China is already making substantial progress with its Grain-for-Green project in the Yellow River basin, conserving soil and water and reducing carbon emissions.

On the flip side, unchecked climate change can worsen erosion. The erosion risk will increase due to emissions driven by temperature changes, decreasing nutrient value and agricultural production. Cultivation without conservation practices is causing soil erosion a hundred times faster than farming.

It has been estimated that global economic losses from soil erosion will be more than $8 billion due to reduced soil fertility, decreased crop yields and increased water usage. At the same time, one report suggests losses of $44 billion annually from erosion.

Results published in Science.org confirm the declines in protein, iron, and zinc and find consistent reductions in vitamins B1, B2, B5, and B9 and, conversely, an increase in vitamin E.

Soil degradation is the decline in soil condition caused by improper use or poor management, usually for agricultural, industrial or urban purposes. It is a severe environmental problem, given that soils are a fundamental natural resource and are the basis for all life.

The soil's original biotic functions of processing nutrients into a form usable by plants have been partially destroyed. Only with significant improvements in farming and soil management can productivity be restored. Farmers need to plough organic matter into the soil a month before planting their crop to improve the soil structure, enhance water and nutrient holding capacity, protect the soil from erosion and compaction, and support a healthy community of soil organisms.

A smaller portion of the world's vegetated land, consisting of 300 million hectares, shows "severe" degradation while its original biotic functions have largely been destroyed. Degradation of less than 1% or 9 million hectares has been classified as "extreme", defined as "unreclaimable and beyond restoration". Its original biotic functions have been destroyed.

According to a new study sponsored by the United Nations Environment Programme (UNEP), an area approximately the size of China and India has suffered moderate to extreme soil degradation caused mainly by agricultural activities, deforestation, and overgrazing in the past forty-five years. This area is 1.2 billion hectares and represents almost 11% of the Earth's vegetated surface.

Seven hundred fifty million hectares of terrain whose degradation is "light", the area with soil degraded just since World War II would be 17% of the Earth's total vegetated land.

Declining Nutrient Composition

A recent study of historical food composition data found apparent declines of between 5% and 40% in some minerals, vitamins, and proteins in groups of vegetables and fruits.

Over 3 billion of the world's population is malnourished in nutrient elements and vitamins. Vegetables and fruits are among the richest sources of many nutrients, so any decline in nutrient concentrations needs to be of great concern.

Ongoing efforts to increase crop yields and apparent tradeoffs between products and the concentrations of half of the essential nutrients work against efforts to increase micronutrients in individual foods.

Micronutrients

There are seven essential plant nutrient elements defined as micronutrients: boron (B), zinc (Zn), manganese (Mn), iron (Fe), copper (Cu), molybdenum (Mo), chlorine (Cl). They constitute less than 1% of the dry weight of most plants.

The water-soluble vitamins with some of their functions are:

- **Vitamin B1 (thiamine):** Helps convert nutrients into energy.
- **Vitamin B2 (riboflavin):** Necessary for energy production, cell function and fat metabolism.
- **Vitamin B3 (niacin):** Drives the production of energy from food.
- **Vitamin B5 (pantothenic acid):** Necessary for the fatty acid synthesis.
- **Vitamin B6 (pyridoxine):** Helps your body release sugar from stored carbohydrates for energy and creates red blood cells.
- **Vitamin B7 (biotin):** Plays a role in the metabolism of fatty acids, amino acids and glucose.
- **Vitamin B9 (folate):** Important for proper cell division.
- **Vitamin B12 (cobalamin):** Necessary for red blood cell formation and maintaining nervous system and brain function.
- **Vitamin C (ascorbic acid):** Required to create neurotransmitters and collagen, the main protein in your skin.

Fat-soluble vitamins do not dissolve in water.

They're best absorbed when consumed alongside a source of fat. After consumption, fat-soluble vitamins are stored in your liver and fatty tissues for future use.

The names and functions of fat-soluble vitamins are:
- **Vitamin A:** Necessary for proper vision and organ function.
- **Vitamin D :** Promotes proper immune function and assists in calcium absorption and bone growth.
- **Vitamin E:** Assists immune function and acts as an antioxidant, protecting cells from damage.
- **Vitamin K:** Required for blood clotting and proper bone development.

The macrominerals and some of their functions are:

- **Calcium:** Necessary for proper structure and function of bones and teeth. Assists in muscle function and blood vessel contraction.
- **Phosphorus:** Part of bone and cell membrane structure.
- **Magnesium:** Assists with over three hundred enzyme reactions, including blood pressure regulation.
- **Sodium:** Electrolyte that aids fluid balance and maintenance of blood pressure.
- **Chloride:** Often found in combination with sodium. It helps maintain fluid balance and is used to make digestive juices.
- **Potassium:** Electrolytes that maintain fluid status in cells and help with nerve transmission and muscle function.
- **Sulphur:** Part of every living tissue and contained in the amino acids methionine and cysteine.

The trace minerals and some of their functions are:

- **Iron:** Helps provide oxygen to muscles and assists in creating certain hormones.
- **Manganese:** Assists in carbohydrate, amino acid and cholesterol metabolism.
- **Copper:** Required for connective tissue formation and normal brain and nervous system function.
- **Zinc:** Necessary for normal growth, immune function and wound healing.
- **Iodine:** Assists in thyroid regulation.
- **Fluoride:** Necessary for the development of bones and teeth.
- **Selenium:** Important for thyroid health, reproduction and defence against oxidative damage.

The Cause of Declining Nutrient Composition

Nutrient depletion of soils is a widespread soil degradation phenomenon due to soil erosion, wind, flood, and poor agricultural practices that do not replenish the nutrients the crops take from the soil.

Common Missing Nutrients in Depleted Soil

The chemical processes determining a soil's fertility are complex, and deficiencies may be difficult to identify. Soils that are heavily fertilised may be rich in macronutrients but very poor in microorganisms and trace minerals. Following are some of the more common minerals missing in today's depleted soils:

Nitrogen

One of the three plant macronutrients, nitrogen leaches quickly from the soil and must be consistently replenished. It must also be in a specific form for plant roots to use. Although commercially added to the soil with ever-increasing fertiliser, nitrogen can remain available throughout all growing seasons through crop rotation, compost, and other soil management techniques.

Calcium

Calcium is essential in a plant's structure and growth. Calcium is returned to the soil through weathered rocks and decaying matter, but modern agriculture, erosion, and acid rain have stripped this mineral away.

Manganese

Vital for photosynthesis and other processes, this micronutrient can become depleted or unavailable to plants when soils are too wet, too high in organic matter, or too high in different elements, such as iron.

Carbon

This element is critical for living microbes to survive. It is used and returned to the soil through organic matter.

GMO Foods

Genetically Modified Food (GMO) is still a relatively new concept and needs further study to determine its impact on health. Science developed GMO foods because of the stress placed on our soil from over farming, the solid declining nutrient value and the commercial gains from increasing the yield of crops.

The most commonly grown GMO foods are corn, soybeans, summer squash, canola, sugar beets, potatoes and papaya.

GMO corn may be found in cornstarch, oil, and processed corn syrup. However, most GMO corn is used to feed livestock like cows and chickens.

About 94% of soybeans are GMOs, but most of the crop is used in animal feed. It's also used to create soybean oil and emulsifiers like soy lecithin and can be found in many processed foods such as cereals, veggie burgers and faux meats, baking mixes, tortillas, granola bars and tofu.

Genetically modified summer squash is resistant to a virus called zucchini yellow mosaic, which can cause severe deformations, blisters, and stunting crop growth.

About 95% of canola that's planted is genetically modified. This crop, used to make canola oil by crushing the seeds, is typically changed to resist herbicides and limit the weeds where it is grown.

More than half of the granulated sugar on supermarket shelves is made from GMO sugar beets.

GMO potatoes are often modified to resist pests and disease and reduce browning and bruising during packaging, transportation, and storage.

The GMO version of this fruit, rainbow papaya, was developed after the ringspot virus.

Summary

The world population is expected to increase from 8.2 billion to 8.5 billion by 2025, and along with this, a growing need for food and water is an issue we will all need to face in the near future.

At the same time, our capacity to grow food with the required nutritional value is declining, forcing us to find supplements to fill this nutritional void.

What does the future hold for us if we cannot produce the quality and quantity of food required to feed the world's growing population?

Like Jules Vern, perhaps Harry Harrison, the author of *Soilent Green*, has the answer.

"In a densely overpopulated, starving New York City of the future, NYPD Detective Robert Thorn (Charlton Heston) investigates the murder of an executive at rations manufacturer Soylent Corporation. With the help of elderly academic Solomon 'Sol' Roth (Edward G. Robinson), Thorn makes real progress—until the governor mysteriously pulls the plug. Obsessed with the mystery, Thorn steps out from behind the badge and launches his investigation into the murder.

"Soylent Green is introduced as made of plankton, but as the film unfolds, the main character discovers it's manufactured from dead bodies. The film's climax contains the line, 'Soylent Green is people!'. This scene is one of the most famous in the movie."

"Climate change raises new challenges for food safety, and effective mitigation includes raising community awareness and promoting and encouraging sustainable practices."

– WHO

Chapter 9
Ground and Surface Water Degradation

Groundwater and surface water are interconnected and can only be managed when understood and acknowledged. If there is a water supply near a source of contamination, that water runs the risk of becoming contaminated. If there is a nearby river or stream, that water can similarly become polluted.

Groundwater can become contaminated from natural sources or residential, municipal, commercial, industrial, and agricultural activities. Contaminants may reach groundwater from activities on the surface, such as spills from stored industrial wastes, sources below the land surface but above the water table, such as septic systems or leaking underground petroleum storage systems.

Millions of fertilisers and pesticides have been used annually for crop production. Farmers, homeowners, businesses, utilities, and municipalities use these chemicals. Many of these entities also use pesticides, which are highly toxic and can enter and contaminate groundwater. Some pesticides remain in the soil and water for months and, in some instances, years.

Water Contaminations

According to The Sydney Morning Herald article on 16 August 2020, "Severe infestations of blue-green algae in Sydney's drinking water catchments have soared 800%, according to an audit which warned climate change is putting the sensitive waterways under increasing threat from toxic blooms."

ABC News reported on 15 March 2021, "Large blooms of toxic blue-green algae in the Murray-Darling Basin and Northern Rivers has prompted Water NSW to issue a red alert health warning for river users and livestock."

As recorded on Wikipedia, *The 1998 Sydney water crisis involved the suspected contamination of the water supply system of Greater Metropolitan*

Sydney by the microscopic pathogens *Cryptosporidium* and *Giardia* between July and September 1998.

Following routine water sampling and testing, over a series of weeks, level contaminants were found at Prospect, Potts Hill, Sydney Hospital, the NSW Art Gallery, Macquarie Street, Centennial Park, Surry Hills, Rhodes, Enfield, Palm Beach, and water treatment facilities at Warragamba, Nepean, North Richmond, Orchard Hills, Woronora, Macarthur, the Illawarra and Prospect. The reliability of these test results was subsequently called into doubt. Precautionary "boil water" alerts were raised, covering several suburban areas for the crisis period.

In response to the crisis, the Government of New South Wales established a Commission of Inquiry, chaired by jurist Peter McClellan QC as Commissioner. McClennan handed down his final report to the NSW Premier, making ninety-one recommendations that led to the reorganisation of water supply and water management functions and agencies in Greater Metropolitan Sydney via the establishment of the Sydney Catchment Authority with responsibility for catchments, dams, and bulk supply reservoirs.

At the same time, Sydney Water managed water supply distribution, water treatment and sewerage, and stormwater management. The Chairman and Managing Director of Sydney Water stood down during and following the crisis.

Residents in Sydney were required to bring their water to a rolling boil for three minutes, subject to elevations above nineteen hundred and eighty metres. Water must be allowed to cool, stored in a clean, sanitised container with a tight cover, and refrigerated.

Sydney Water now claims water is filtered to the high standards set by the Australian Drinking Water Guidelines, ensuring it's safe to drink straight from the tap. "Greater Sydney has some of the best drinking water globally".

These changes have marked improvement in the quality of our drinking water and established management guidelines to minimise and hopefully eliminate problems like this from ever happening again.

From the Reservoir to the Tap

Houses built during the 1960s and earlier were often equipped with galvanised sewer and water pipe systems and were coated in a layer of zinc to extend their effective lifespan. Today, galvanised piping can cause several problems for water quality regardless of the quality Sydney Water claims to deliver.

Naturally occurring zinc, used in constructing galvanised pipes, contains several impurities, such as lead and iron. Over decades of usage, the water that passes through these pipes slowly corrodes the walls of galvanised piping, allowing small deposits of iron and other minerals to separate from the zinc interior and build up in the water itself.

Lead poisoning occurs when lead builds up in the body, often over months or years; even small amounts of information can cause serious health problems. Children younger than six years are especially vulnerable to lead poisoning, severely affecting mental and physical development, while high lead levels can be fatal.

That aside, Sydney Water claims, "We add a small amount of chlorine to your drinking water at our filtration plants to protect you from microorganisms. Chlorine is safe and effective. The amounts we add are informed by the Australian Drinking Water Guidelines. We try to minimise the taste and smell of chlorine in your drinking water. Let your water stand in a jug or put it in the fridge overnight if you notice it."

Acquiring a water filtration and purification system for the water consumed has become a priority for many Australians, as it has for people worldwide.

Water filters deliver the highest quality of drinking water using a carbon block filter to reduce more than hundred and forty possible contaminants, including lead, pesticides, chlorine, and mercury, by trapping them in the carbon block filter while leaving nearly 100% of beneficial minerals such as calcium, magnesium and fluoride in the water. Plus, use an ultra-violet technology that delivers 80 millijoules of UV light to destroy more than 99.99% of undesirable bacteria and viruses in your drinking water.

Apart from anything else, the taste test alone will confirm the difference between the quality of the water delivered via the tap and the water passed through a filtering solution that meets the abovementioned requirement.

Water Contamination and Required Treatments

Drinking water sources are subject to contamination and require treatments to remove germs, minerals, and other waterborne particles. The most common steps in water treatment used by water management departments for surface water include:

Coagulation and Flocculation

Coagulation and flocculation are often the first steps in water treatment. Let me tell you, without the full technical description of how this process works, the same technology is used when your swimming pool is full of suspended matter. Flock is added and circulated for some time; circulation is then stopped. The flock binds with all suspended materials, falls to the bottom of the pool, and is vacuumed to waste. Not through the filter because running flock through a filter during circulation or vacuuming will kill the filter.

Sedimentation

Due to its weight, flock settles to the bottom of the water supply during sedimentation.

Filtration

Once the flock has settled to the bottom of the water supply, the clear water on top passes through filters of varying compositions, including compacted sand, gravel, and charcoal, each with different pore sizes, to remove dissolved particles, such as dust, parasites, bacteria, viruses, and chemicals.

Disinfection

After the water has been filtered, disinfectants like chlorine and chloramine may be added to kill any remaining parasites, bacteria, and viruses and protect the water from germs when piped to homes and businesses.

Water Ratios in the Human Body

Considering water makes up 73% of our brain and heart, 79% of our muscles and kidneys, and 92% of our blood is water, it stands to reason that the water we consume should be of the highest possible quality.

Summary

As drinking water becomes more scarce, governments worldwide will be forced to treat ground and surface water more aggressively. Some locations have already turned to storage treatment to provide drinking water as the only available water for consumption.

Of course, we can purchase bottled spring water, but the cost exceeds the cost of petrol per litre, which may be cost-prohibitive for most people.

(According to the Food and Drug Administration, spring water must come from an underground source and flow naturally to the earth's surface. But *spring water doesn't have to be collected at the spring*—it can also be pumped out from a hole in the ground.)

The alternative to buying bottled spring or filtered water is to purchase your drinking water filtering system.

"Like air, water is fundamental to life itself. We need it to survive and thrive."

– WHO

Chapter 10
Nutrition

The world grows 95% of its food in the uppermost layer of soil, making topsoil one of the most critical components of our food system. Over half of that soil has disappeared in the last century because of our conventional farming practices and wind and water erosion, which have contributed to a decline in the nutrient value of crops.

Nutrient pollution has impacted our streams, rivers, lakes, bays and coastal waters for several decades, resulting in severe environmental and human health issues and impacting the economy. Too much nitrogen and phosphorus in the water cause algae to grow faster than ecosystems can handle.

On the other side of this problem, people like Norman Borlaug (PhD in Pathology and Genetics) were awarded the Nobel Peace Prize for his contributions to the world food supply in 1970. Borlaug continually advocated increasing crop yields as a means to curb deforestation. Promoting this view led to this methodology being called by agricultural economists the "Borlaug hypothesis", namely that increasing the productivity of agriculture on the best farmland can help control deforestation by reducing the demand for new farmland.

Borlaug believed that global food demand was on the rise and that restricting crops to traditional low-yield methods would require the world population to decrease, either voluntarily or due to mass starvation or the conversion of forest land into cropland. It is thus argued that high-yield techniques are ultimately saving ecosystems from destruction.

Borlaug's new semi-dwarf, disease-resistant varieties, called Pitic 62 and Penjamo 62, changed the potential yield of spring wheat dramatically. By 1963, 95% of Mexico's wheat crops used the semi-dwarf varieties developed by Borlaug. That year, the harvest was six times larger than in 1944, when Borlaug arrived in Mexico. Mexico had become fully self-sufficient in wheat production and a net wheat exporter.

Food; Quality; Nutrition; Balance

A balanced diet comprises carbohydrates, protein, and fats; mixing these core food groups in any diet should be carefully considered.

Carbohydrates are integral for protein tissue synthesis and are stored in our muscles to govern energy production, speed, concentration, stamina, and fluid balance.

Dietary carbohydrates can be segmented into the following three classifications:

Sugars

Sugars are carbohydrates that occur naturally in many foods but are also added as ingredients and used by the body for energy.

Simple sugars are monosaccharides, including glucose (dextrose), fructose, and galactose.

The sugar most commonly used as table sugar is sucrose. This sugar is a disaccharide broken down in the body into fructose and glucose for energy.

There is very little difference between the types of sugar you find in the supermarket (e.g., white, brown, raw, etc.). They are different because of the other processing techniques used in their manufacture.

Experts generally agree that eating excess kilojoules contributes to weight gain. Being overweight or obese increases the risk of chronic health problems like high blood pressure, type-2 diabetes and heart disease.

Sugar provides the same amount of energy or kilojoules (kJ) per gram as other digestible carbohydrates such as starch in bread, rice and pasta.

The World Health Organisation (WHO) recommends that "free" sugars make up no more than 10% of daily kilojoule intake to prevent unhealthy weight gain and dental caries.

Starches

Starch is the most common carbohydrate in the human diet and contains many staple foods. The significant sources of starch intake worldwide are cereals (rice, wheat, and maize) and root vegetables (potatoes and cassava).

Widely used foods containing starch are bread, pancakes, cereals, noodles, pasta, porridge and tortillas.

Digestive enzymes have problems digesting crystalline structures. Raw starch is digested poorly in the duodenum and small intestine, while bacterial degradation occurs mainly in the colon. When starch is cooked, the digestibility is increased.

Before the advent of processed foods, people consumed large amounts of uncooked and unprocessed starch-containing plants, which contained high amounts of resistant starch. Microbes within the large intestine ferment the starch to produce short-chain fatty acids, which are used as energy and support the maintenance and growth of the microbes.

More highly processed foods are easily digested and release more glucose in the small intestine, while less starch reaches the large intestine, and the body absorbs more energy.

Starch can be classified as rapidly digestible, slowly digestible and resistant starch. Raw starch granules resist digestion by human enzymes and do not break down into glucose in the small intestine—they reach the large intestine and function as prebiotic dietary fibre.

Fibre

Dietary fibre is found mainly in fruits, vegetables, whole grains, and legumes and is best known for preventing or relieving constipation.

Foods containing fibre can provide other health benefits, such as helping maintain a healthy weight and lowering your risk of diabetes, heart disease and cancer.

Whole carbs or simple carbs refer to unprocessed carbohydrates containing fibre found naturally in food; think fruits, legumes, potatoes, and whole grains.

Refined carbs, alternatively known as complex carbs, are stripped of fibre.

Proteins are often called the building blocks of tissue and are composed of amino acids and break down in the body to form muscle mass and metabolic regulation.

Some great protein sources include natural peanut butter, eggs, quinoa, edamame, plain Greek yoghurt, black beans, and sunflower seeds.

Dietary Fats provide our bodies with energy and support cell growth. There are four main classifications of fats in the food we eat.

Saturated Fats

Saturated fats can cause problems with cholesterol levels, increasing your risk of heart disease. Saturated fats are found in animal-based foods like beef, pork, poultry, full-fat dairy products, eggs, and tropical oils like coconut and palm. Because they are typically solid at room temperature and sometimes called "solid fats".

Unsaturated Fats

They are referred to as "good fats" and are preferred by most health professionals, but they are needed as with most things consumed in moderation.

Found in meats, lard, and dairy products; trans fats are found in packaged baked goods, potato chips and fast food. Monosaturated fats are found most conveniently in nuts and seeds, and Polyunsaturated fats, an abundance of which are found in fish, seed oils and oysters.

Monounsaturated Fats

Monounsaturated fatty acids, or MUFAs, are a type of unsaturated fat. "Mono", meaning one, signifies that monounsaturated fats have only one double bond and can be found in olive, peanut, and canola oils, avocados, nuts such as almonds, hazelnuts, and pecans and seeds such as pumpkin and sesame seeds.

Polyunsaturated Fats

Polyunsaturated fats are usually liquid at room temperature and are called "oils". They're found mainly in Sunflower, corn, soybean, flaxseed oils, walnuts, flax seeds, fish, and canola oil, though higher in monounsaturated fat; they are also a good source of polyunsaturated fat; omega-3 fats are an essential type of polyunsaturated fat.

Sugar

Sugars are carbohydrates that occur naturally in many foods but are also added as ingredients and used by the body for energy.

Simple sugars are monosaccharides, including glucose (dextrose), fructose, and galactose.

The sugar most commonly used as table sugar is sucrose. This sugar is a disaccharide broken down in the body into fructose and glucose for energy.

There is very little difference between the types of sugar you find in the supermarket (e.g., white, brown, raw, etc.). They are different because of the other processing techniques used in their manufacture.

Experts generally agree that eating excess kilojoules contributes to weight gain. Being overweight or obese increases the risk of chronic health problems like high blood pressure, type-2 diabetes and heart disease.

Sugar provides the same amount of energy or kilojoules (kJ) per gram as other digestible carbohydrates such as starch in bread, rice and pasta.

The World Health Organisation (WHO) recommends that "free" sugars make up no more than 10% of daily kilojoule intake to prevent unhealthy weight gain and dental caries.

While the argument for eliminating or reducing sugar consumption from our diets rages, we must consider a straightforward fact first.

To eliminate added sugars from our diets, we first need to find them, which is no easy feat. Sugar goes by many names, including agave, brown sugar, cane sugar, coconut palm sugar, evaporated cane juice, fruit juice concentrate (apple or pear juice concentrate), honey, brown rice maple syrup and high-fructose corn syrup.

While our food labelling standards vary considerably from country to country, we see distinctions between the naturally occurring ones and those added.

Sugar Substitutes

Artificial sweeteners trigger the same sensory cells in our taste buds that send signals to our brains when we taste something sweet, like sugar. Because artificial sweeteners are between two hundred and twenty thousand times sweeter than sugar, manufacturers can use so little to add almost no calories in their formulation.

The following list of artificial sweeteners is all approved for use in foods.

- Saccharin
- Aspartame
- Acesulfame potassium (Ace-K)
- Sucralose
- Neotame
- Advantame
- Steviol glycosides
- Luo Han Guo fruit extracts

High-intensity sweeteners are commonly used as sugar substitutes or alternatives because they are often sweeter than sugar but contribute only a few to no calories when added to foods.

Junk Food

Junk food, or perhaps we should label it "Convenience Food" in many instances, lacks the nutrients, vitamins, and minerals our bodies need and is high in kilojoules (energy), salts, sugars, and fats.

Some examples of junk food include:

- cakes and biscuits
- fast foods (such as hot chips, burgers and pizzas)
- chocolate and sweets
- processed meat (such as bacon)
- snacks (such as chips)
- sugary drinks (such as sports, energy and soft drinks)
- alcoholic drinks

While reducing the amount of junk food you eat can be challenging, you don't have to give up on your favourite foods.

Plan your meals and snacks, so you decide what you eat based on nutrition, not what is left in your pantry. Planning also helps you keep to a budget and makes shopping more manageable.

- Choose wholefood options such as wholemeal and wholegrain carbohydrates like pasta, bread, and flour.

- Choose fresh fruit for dessert instead of junk food to avoid added salt, sugar and saturated fat.
- Check your food's nutritional value using the nutritional information panel on the back of the packet.
- Watch out for foods that claim to be reduced in fat (having less fat than the previous version doesn't mean they aren't still high in fat).

A Balanced Diet

A balanced diet comprises carbohydrates, protein, and fats; mixing these core food groups in any diet should be carefully considered.

The Ratio of Carbs, Protein & Fat

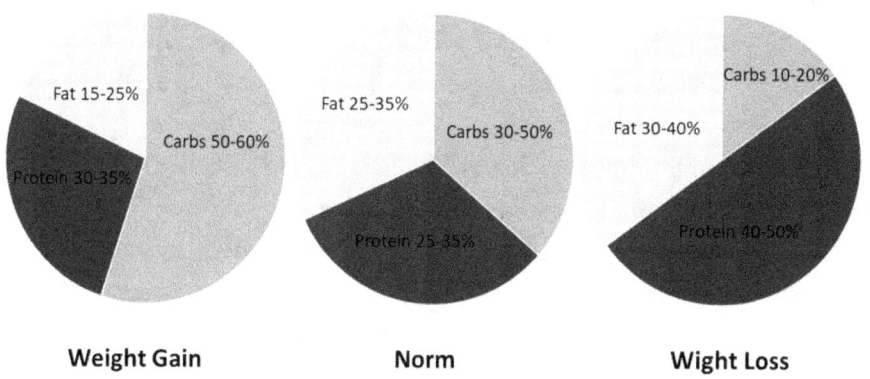

| Weight Gain | Norm | Wight Loss |

A balanced diet is a diet that contains differing kinds of foods in specific quantities and proportions so that the requirement for calories, proteins, minerals, vitamins and alternative nutrients is adequate.

The table above should clarify that weight gain is inevitable with high carbohydrate (sugar) intake. In contrast, carbohydrate reduction is associated with weight loss.

Summary

Eat healthily; what does that mean these days? Well, I think the message here, from my perspective, is to eat less sugar and processed or manufactured food and instead eat more protein, vegetables and fruit.

Our lifestyle has changed over the last hundred years from longer working hours with higher levels of physical activity to a screen-based environment that is more sedentary. I see this daily with my children, their husbands, and friends constantly scrolling through their phones. Sure, we live in a world where information is at our fingertips any time of the day and night, and it's almost impossible to disengage from email and social media.

The price of this lifestyle change became very apparent with COVID-19 and our switch to ordering food via DoorDash, UberEats, and many more apps that allow cooked food to be delivered directly to the front door of your house. Over the past eighteen months, these food delivery services have satisfied my three daughters and their partners' daily and night desires.

Processed food high in fats and sugar combined with screen-based activity and online university study changed our engagement with food. It will continue to impact our choices for many years to come.

My wife and I have resisted these services for the last eighteen months. We consume various foods from the five major food groups, providing different nutrients to our bodies, promoting good health and reducing disease risk. We also lost almost 40 kilograms because we ate the right foods, with the right balance of fats, carbohydrates and proteins.

Fats and oils are high in kilojoules but necessary for a healthy diet in small amounts.

No matter where you're starting, it's easy to make minor changes while focusing on eating foods from the five major food groups and reducing your processed and manufactured foods intake.

"The doctor of the future will no longer treat the human frame with drugs, but rather will cure and prevent disease with nutrition."

– Thomas Edison

"Let food be thy medicine and medicine be thy food."

– Hippocrates

Chapter 11
Supplementation

The research outlined in Chapter 8 shows a significant decline in the nutritional value of food, plus the ground and surface water degradation summarised in Chapter 9, which is evidence of why everyone should take supplements.

I take the following supplements daily to ensure my nutritional requirements are met. I also take a few additional supplements to aid arthritis and bone-on-bone condition of my knees and cardiovascular disease.

The omega-3 and the glucosamine have made it possible to walk the distances I do daily. In contrast, magnesium has enabled my leg muscles to recover quickly from the distances I walk daily and eliminate my leg cramps at night.

Probiotic

Replaces the good bacteria lost in your gut from stress, pollution or unhealthy eating with 6.3 billion live probiotic microorganisms (per serve) from five strains, including two of the most well-studied probiotic strains (Lactobacilli and Bifidobacteria), to help support a healthy digestive and immune system.

Bacteria is usually viewed negatively as something that makes you sick. However, you constantly have two kinds of bacteria in and on your body—good and harmful. Probiotics combine beneficial bacteria and yeasts that naturally live in your body. Probiotics are made up of good bacteria that help keep your body healthy and working well. This good bacteria helps you in many ways, including fighting off harmful bacteria when you have too much of it, helping you feel better.

Omega-3

Omega-3 Complex is a natural fish oil supplement from cold-water fish to help you become a well-oiled machine. Each capsule contains essential fatty acids not naturally manufactured by the body—omega-3 assists in maintaining a healthy heart and normal blood cholesterol levels.

Omega-3 fatty acids help all the cells in your body function as they should. They're a vital part of your cell membranes, helping to provide structure and supporting interactions between cells. While they're essential to all your cells, omega-3s are concentrated in your eyes and brain cells.

In addition, omega-3s provide your body with energy (calories) and support the health of many body systems. These include your cardiovascular system and endocrine system.

Multi-Vitamin

Multi-vitamin, multi-mineral, and phytonutrient supplements offer a comprehensive and balanced range of nutrients. It contains twelve essential vitamins, ten essential minerals, and twenty-two plant concentrates from fruits, vegetables and herb extracts representing all five colours of the phytonutrient spectrum.

There are thirteen essential vitamins your body needs for normal, healthy functioning.

Nutrients are substances used by living things to survive and grow. These are nutrients your body cannot make itself (or cannot make enough of). It must get most of them through diet.

Vitamins are usually only needed in small amounts. Too much of some can cause symptoms or toxicity.

A healthy diet provides all the nutrients, including the thirteen essential vitamins. Poor health and illness can occur when vitamins are missing from the diet. For example, scurvy is caused by a shortage of vitamin C, and rickets is caused by a long-term vitamin D deficiency.

Cal-Mag D

Advanced is a mineral supplement that supplies calcium, magnesium, and vitamin D for a balanced approach to supplementation, providing additional calcium and magnesium that may be lacking in the diet. This advanced formula, along with a healthy diet and physical activity, may assist with preventing osteoporosis later in life.

Of all the essential minerals in your body, calcium is the most abundant. Nearly all of your calcium is stored in your bones and teeth.

Like magnesium, calcium is vital to bone health. It enables bones to develop and grow, keeping them strong and dense until around twenty-five. After twenty-five, your bones lose density as part of the ageing process. Calcium helps slow this decline.

Calcium also contributes to establishing:

- Muscle function
- Blood clotting
- Neurotransmission (nerve cells passing signals to each other)
- Digestive enzyme function

Siberian Ginseng and Ginkgo Biloba

Siberian Ginseng and Ginkgo Biloba Blend tackles stamina, stress, and energy. It is a natural way to deal with the rigours of high activity and stress by targeting the adrenal glands to allow your body to handle stress better. Traditionally, Ginkgo has been used to maintain blood flow to the body's extremities and may help maintain memory function.

Siberian ginseng is often called an "adaptogen". This non-medical term describes substances that can supposedly strengthen the body and increase general resistance to daily stress.

In addition to being an adaptogen, Siberian ginseng is used for heart and blood vessel conditions, such as high blood pressure, low blood pressure, hardening of the arteries, and rheumatic heart disease.

It is also used for kidney disease, Alzheimer's disease, attention deficit-hyperactivity disorder (ADHD), chronic fatigue syndrome, diabetes, high cholesterol, improving the loss of sensation in extremities (peripheral neuropathy), fibromyalgia, rheumatoid arthritis, reducing the effects of a hangover, flu, colds, chronic bronchitis, and tuberculosis. It is also used to treat the side effects of chemotherapy.

Siberian ginseng improves athletic performance and treats sleep problems (insomnia) and the symptoms of infections caused by herpes simplex type-2.

It also boosts the immune system, prevents colds, and increases appetite.

Concentrated Fruits and Vegetables

The formula contains rich sources of nutrients, antioxidants and phytonutrients that assist your body in maintaining optimal health. This phytonutrient-based supplement also helps to minimise the harmful effects of free radicals from lifestyles such as pollution, stress, smoking and irregular diet.

Vitamin C Plus

Vitamin C Plus tackles allergies, flu, and colds head-on. One tablet of Vitamin C Plus Extended Release provides the body with 500mg of vitamin C slowly and gently throughout the day, ensuring it is always available as needed.

Vitamin C is a powerful antioxidant that can strengthen your body's natural defences.

Antioxidants are molecules that boost the immune system. They do so by protecting cells from harmful molecules called free radicals. When free radicals accumulate, they can promote a state known as oxidative stress, which has been linked to many chronic diseases.

Studies show that consuming more vitamin C can increase your blood antioxidant levels by up to 30%, helping the body's natural defences fight inflammation.

Glucosamine HCl with Boswellia

Glucosamine HCl with Boswellia supports joint health by helping reduce joint swelling and increase mobility caused by osteoarthritis.

One of its leading roles is to support the healthy development of articular cartilage, a type of smooth white tissue that covers the ends of your bones where they meet to form joints.

Along with the lubricating liquid called synovial fluid, articular cartilage minimises friction and allows bones to move freely and painlessly across one another.

Glucosamine promotes the creation of certain chemical compounds, including collagen, essential structural components of articular cartilage and synovial fluid.

Some studies indicate that taking glucosamine supplements may protect joint tissue by preventing the breakdown of cartilage, particularly in athletes.

CoQ10

Coenzyme (CoQ10) is an antioxidant that supports heart health and boosts your body's natural energy while protecting body cells from free radical damage.

As we age, the levels of CoQ10 in our bodies decrease. CoQ10 is lower in people with certain conditions, such as heart disease, and those who take cholesterol-lowering drugs called statins.

As dietary supplements, CoQ10 is available in capsules, chewable tablets, liquid syrups, wafers, and IVs. CoQ10 is believed to help prevent or treat certain heart conditions and migraine headaches.

Research on CoQ10 use for specific conditions and activities shows:

- **Heart conditions:** CoQ10 has been shown to improve symptoms of congestive heart failure. Although findings are mixed, CoQ10 might help reduce blood pressure. Some research also suggests that CoQ10 might aid recovery in people with bypass and heart valve surgeries when combined with other nutrients.
- **Diabetes:** Although more studies are needed, some research suggests that CoQ10 may help reduce low-density lipoprotein (LDL) cholesterol and total cholesterol levels in people with diabetes, lowering their risk of heart disease.
- **Parkinson's disease:** Recent research suggests that even high doses of CoQ10 don't seem to improve symptoms in people with Parkinson's.
- **Statin-induced myopathy:** Some research suggests that CoQ10 might help ease muscle weakness and pain sometimes associated with statins.

Magnesium

Magnesium is a helpful and convenient way to support normal muscle function, electrolyte balance, and bone health. Plus, it can also help to reduce tiredness and fatigue.

Magnesium plays many crucial roles in the body, such as supporting muscle and nerve function and energy production.

Low magnesium levels usually don't cause symptoms. However, chronically low levels can increase the risk of high blood pressure, heart disease, type-2 diabetes and osteoporosis.

As a sufferer of peripheral neuropathy caused by type-2 diabetes, the nerves in my legs and arms were severely damaged, resulting in acute nerve pain, muscle atrophy and being numb from the waist down. I have used magnesium supplements to promote nerve regeneration and help rebuild the muscles in my legs in combination with walking long distances daily.

While I still experience balance issues in the dark, I have full sensations in my legs and a vastly improved feeling in my feet. In addition, I have eliminated pain medication from my list of prescriptions.

Summary

Suppose you have decided to switch to eating primarily healthy and whole foods, reduce your stress levels, up your exercise program, and get a better quality of sleep. In that case, you may believe these lifestyle changes will be enough to reclaim your health. While these changes will unquestionably improve your health and help you lose weight, the nutritional value of the food you eat and the quality of the water you drink is not the same as it was for the previous generation.

Nutritional supplementation is designed to fill the void created by the declining quality of the food and water our bodies require. They can dramatically improve our vitality, help us live healthier lifestyles, and improve our quality of life.

While a whole foods diet should provide you with all the vitamins and nutrients needed for optimum health, our environment and lifestyle choices make it much more complicated than it was for our ancestors.

In the past, harvests fully embodied the vital nutrients of the soil and sea, nourishing people. In essence, our fishing and farming methods have changed drastically. With the combination of modern intensive farming methods, our modern lifestyles and the urban environments we live in, it is necessary to consider adding supplements to your health regime for many reasons.

Many nutritional supplements have been proven to prevent or aid in treating health conditions like high cholesterol, arthritis, congenital disabilities, and cancer.

In Chapter 8, I outlined the significant decline in the nutritional value of food; in combination with the ground and surface water degradation summarised in Chapter 9, the nutrients in our product have not been allowed to replenish in the soil naturally.

Organic farmers have introduced hybrid crops because of the increased yield per acre, which has resulted in lower nutrient content.

Farmers once used manure for fertilisers; today, they use superphosphate fertilisers that contain nitrogen, potassium and phosphorus but are deficient in many other nutrients.

Pesticides and herbicides damage the soil microorganisms needed to make minerals and other nutrients available to plants; when lacking, the food is often much lower in nutrient content.

Food processing and refining techniques reduce the nutrient content of the wheat used to make white flour, removing over 80% of its magnesium, 70% of its zinc, 80% of its chromium, 80% of its manganese, and 50% of its cobalt while polishing rice removes about over 70% of its zinc and chromium.

Artificial flavours, colours, stabilisers, and preservatives added to food may even increase the quality of food by preserving it; many are toxic and can deplete the nutrient value of the food.

Micronutrients (minerals and vitamins) play a significant part in good health. The number of minerals and vitamins we need may be small compared to macronutrients such as proteins, carbohydrates and fats, but their influence on our well-being is profound.

If, after reading this book and researching the decline in the nutritional value of food and ground and surface water degradation, you are still not convinced about the importance of taking supplements because your body has adjusted to the new sub-normal.

Try taking supplements for thirty days, and if you don't find a dramatic increase in energy and vitality, I will walk down George Street in Sydney backwards and naked.

"Getting all the nutrients you need simply cannot be done without supplements."

– Steven Gundry

Chapter 12
Weight Management

Choices It's All About Choices

Health is a choice, but for most people, it's more about what we have come to accept rather than fighting to achieve or maintain.

Global statistics prove this point.

According to the Australian Government, a day in our nation's health in 2018 looks like the following.

- eighty-five babies are born
- four hundred and forty people die
- three hundred and eighty people are diagnosed with cancer
- hundred and seventy people experience a heart attack
- hundred people have a stroke
- fourteen people are newly diagnosed with end-stage kidney disease
- thirteen hundred people are hospitalised due to injury

Indicator	Australia's ranking out of thirty-five countries	Australia's relative position
Indicators grouped as best/middle/worst		
Life expectancy, males	5	Best third
Life expectancy, females	8	Best third
Coronary heart disease mortality	17	Middle third
Dementia prevalence	17	Middle third
Daily smoking	6	Best third

Alcohol consumption	21	Middle third
Obesity	30	Worst third
Colon cancer survival	3	Best third

Basic Regulation of Eating and Body Weight

The body is in a continual state of hunger, intermittently relieved by eating. This perpetual drive to eat is suppressed by inhibitory impulses generated by food in the gastrointestinal tract, the flow of nutrients into the blood and other factors. After these "satiety factors" have dissipated, the desire to eat returns.

Weight

Several things help determine a person's weight, including genes and hormones. Your body holds on to extra calories and turns them into fat. But being overweight or obese usually comes from eating the wrong food or more than is required.

So there are two things you must change to lose weight in a healthy and lasting way:

- Eat right
- Move more

BMI

BMI uses weight and height to determine whether an adult is within the healthy weight range, underweight, overweight or obese.

It estimates total body fat as a proportion of body weight and the risk of developing weight-related diseases.

BMI is calculated by dividing weight by the height square: BMI = Weight (kg)/Height (m)2.

When calculating your BMI, measuring your weight in kilograms and your height in centimetres is essential.

To find your weight classification (if you are an adult), see which of these BMI ranges your weight falls into:

- Under 18.5: underweight
- 18.5-24.9: healthy weight range

- 25.0-29.9: overweight
- 30.0 and above: obese

Fat

Fat comprises a single lipid droplet with far fewer mitochondria; white fat has a lighter white or yellow appearance. It is the predominant form of fat in the body. It has several purposes, including being the most significant energy reserve in the body, a thermal insulator and cushion for our internal organs, and just being a big cushion, protecting us when we inevitably bump into things. White fat is also a major endocrine organ, producing oestrogen and leptin, which helps regulate appetite and hunger.

Visceral Fat

Visceral fat is stored in a person's abdominal cavity and is known as "active fat" as it influences how hormones function. Therefore, an excess of visceral fat can have potentially dangerous consequences.

Because visceral fat is in the abdominal cavity, it is close to many vital organs, such as the pancreas, liver, and intestines.

The more visceral fat a person stores, the more at risk for certain health complications, such as type-2 diabetes and heart disease.

Fast facts on visceral fat:

- Excess visceral fat can cause serious health problems
- Exercising for a minimum of 30 minutes each day will help burn visceral fat
- Having some amount of body fat is perfectly healthy and normal

Body Age

Body Age calculators are frequently used in health publications by gyms and personal trainers to set achievable targets for people wanting to improve their health and fitness. In essence, they help reduce the metabolic age and fitness age.

Almost without exception, these body age calculators show the person being tested has a "biological age" that is older than it should be.

All these age calculators compare your measurements for a range of health risk factors to an average or an ideal number to determine your score. Having an older biological age on these calculators means you have at least one risk factor higher than the number set as "normal".

But unless we know which specific risk factors are above average and how normal they are defined, it's hard to see if you should be worried or what you should do about it.

Muscle Mass

Muscle mass is challenging to measure. It also depends on many factors, including height, ethnicity, and fitness level.

The following charts are based on this study. While new research is necessary, this data will give you an idea of muscle mass percentages for different age groups.

Muscle mass percentage averages for men:

Age	Muscle mass percentage
18-35	40-44
36-55	36-40
56-75	32-35
76-85	<31

Muscle mass percentage averages for women:

Age	Muscle mass percentage
18-35	31-33
36-55	29-31
56-75	27-30
76-85	<26

Overweight and Obesity

The effects of being overweight or obese are significant. If you think you are overweight, your BMI is higher than 30.0, or you are obese, you risk developing serious complications that will shorten your life or reduce the quality of your life.

I know because I lived in denial most of my life. The consequences of that denial have caused me considerable difficulties and more continuous pain than most people would be capable of bearing.

Listed below are the health conditions that can occur due to being overweight. The items shown in red are conditions for which I have been under treatment.

- All causes of death (mortality)
- High blood pressure (Hypertension)
- High LDL cholesterol, low HDL cholesterol, or high levels of triglycerides (Dyslipidemia)
- Type-1 and 2 diabetes
- Peripheral Neuropathy (Numb from the waist down)
- Coronary heart disease
- Stroke
- Kidney disease
- Gallbladder disease
- Osteoarthritis (a breakdown of cartilage and bone within a joint)
- Sleep apnoea and breathing problems
- Low quality of life
- Mental illnesses such as clinical depression, anxiety, and other mental disorders
- Body pain and difficulty with physical functioning

I have overcome the effects of being overweight and obese and avoided the first item on the list, albeit only just. I have been able to reverse the following conditions:

- High blood pressure (Hypertension)
- High LDL cholesterol, low HDL cholesterol, or high levels of triglycerides (Dyslipidemia)
- Type-2 diabetes
- Peripheral Neuropathy (Numb from the waist down)
- Kidney disease
- Low quality of life
- Mental illnesses such as clinical depression, anxiety, and other mental disorders

The most significant of these has been the regeneration of nerve sensation in my legs and feet. I am no longer numb from the waist down, and I have eliminated Lyrica I was taking for the nerve pain in my legs and feet.

Healthy Weight Management

Almost anyone who follows readily available diets can achieve and maintain a healthy weight. Maintaining that healthy weight for the rest of your life requires a commitment to changing the habits of a lifetime. If this were not so, the habits that brought you to the point requiring your commitment and action would not be an issue.

Healthy eating, physical activity, optimal sleep, and stress reduction are essential to any weight loss program. Still, just as importantly, we need to retrain our thinking and understand that our habits are the key to losing the extra weight and keeping that weight off for the rest of our lives.

Healthy eating is not just eating healthy foods or stopping fast/convenient high-fat, high-sugar foods and drinks; it's about cutting sugar and processed foods from your diet and eating consistently throughout the day.

Fad diets may promise fast results, but such diets limit your nutritional intake, can be unhealthy, and tend to fail in the long run.

The physical activity required to balance your changed dietary intake need not be excessive. Still, the time you undertake this activity and its intensity will go a long way to helping you lose those extra kilograms and keep them off.

Walking briskly, given this, will vary for men and women based on age, and the additional weight they carry will differ. But a good rule of thumb is that anything that doubles your resting heart rate is ideal.

Managing your weight is never top of mind; it wasn't from my perspective. Looking back over family photographs from the past thirty years, it's not hard to see the extra weight I was carrying or why it contributed to the onset of diabetes.

As I have said, the title of this book explains, "Life is a Gift, Health is a Choice", and those "Choices have Consequences". Sometimes, those consequences result in unrepairable damage to your body, which doesn't become apparent until after the damage has been done.

Summary

At this point, it should be evident from all the statistics on obesity that health is dramatically influenced by being overweight. Still, as you will see in later chapters, I talk about why the traditional methods we use to reduce or manage weight don't work, or if they do, the effect is only temporary.

There is no such thing as weight management; forget everything you have ever heard about weight management. Health is your life and the only thing you need to manage.

Race car drivers talk about not looking at the wall at the next corner because what you are looking at is what you will hit.

Look at your health instead; focus on everything you have to reduce or eliminate, your doctor's medication to control your medical conditions. Focus on dropping the number of specialists you have to see regularly and try to find a local family doctor who cares enough about you rather than how much time you spend with them compared to the service fee they have been able to charge.

Start small simply by walking around the block once every morning, and as you build strength, walk around it twice, take the stairs instead of the escalator, walk to the shops instead of driving and remember it is the activity that will help you improve your health.

The hardest thing in the world to overcome is its inertia, and it's evident that it is easier to keep moving once inertia has been overcome.

"Your current body is the only body that can take you to your new body, so be kind to it."

– Elaine Moran

Chapter 13
Mental Health

The one lesson we have learnt from the COVID-19 pandemic is *that we are social animals, and any form of incarceration is unnatural for us as a species.*

Being forced to isolate if you live alone is no different than being forced to separate in a house filled with people.

Our mental health requires a certain amount of freedom to do what we want when we want to do it and move around when needed. Our house was full of people: my wife, two of our daughters, husband and partner, and Jacqui's sister, albeit temporarily, and getting time on your own can be just as troubling as not being able to spend time in the company of others.

As a sufferer of depression and to the extent that I tried to take my life in 2014, I think I can qualify as a person with skin in the game. While the lessons from that episode are still vivid in my mind, it is also reasonable to say that I still struggle with depression.

I still remember my first counselling session and how I determined I needed to do "whatever I have to do or say to get me out of here attitude" due to my psychologist's psychoanalysing. The hardest part of the process was that I didn't want to talk about the issue that took me to the edge, and I realised that unless I gave him what he needed to assess me and believed I was OK, I would never get the all-clear.

So I told him what he needed to hear, stringing it out over several weeks and multiple sessions.

After planning my second suicide and being found out, I was pushed back to a second psychologist. The very different approach, given that I didn't want to talk, he just sat there to read a book, occasionally lifting his head to see what I was doing before returning to his book.

At the end of the first session, he said, "I am here to listen, and when you are ready to talk, we can look at ways to help you, but until then, you're paying me to read my book".

We connected because he played me the same way I played my previous psychologist, so I started to open up to him about what was troubling me, and he just listened. After several weeks of listening came questions, and from my answers, more questions helped me realise he was interested only in helping me.

I tell you this story because I know from my perspective that I never wanted to talk about myself or my issues, which is why the method my psychologist gave me to help me deal with my depression helped me then. I still use it today when I experience my darker moments.

Finding someone interested in you who is willing to listen when the last thing you want to do is talk is essential for anyone who suffers from depression. Leaning there is no way out of your depression unless you slowly talk it out with someone who has earned your trust is the first step to helping you find your way.

Young Adults and Mental Health

Just like other illnesses, mental illnesses need to be managed. If you think you could have a mental health issue or know someone you love or care for is experiencing mental health issues, consider getting help.

Young adults experience the same mental health issues as adults, plus a few additional generational pressures.

The following is not a complete list of mental health issues, but it's a good starting point for discussion:

- feel stressed
- have relationship issues
- have financial worries
- develop a drug or alcohol problem
- struggle with work or study
- need help looking after a child
- have low self-esteem
- feel too fat or too skinny
- experience bullying at work or online

It doesn't necessarily mean your mental health is in danger if you're having a tough time with these or other issues. But reaching out to someone and discussing your problems is a good start.

If you are thinking about self-harm or suicide, you need to reach out and find some help.

Alternatively, you can learn more about your issue and get help by:

- talking to your friends and family
- eating well, getting enough sleep
- get some regular exercise
- make time to relax and have some fun
- if you're using drugs or alcohol, cut down or stop

Finally, you may be upset if the people you thought would understand your situation and who you contacted for help let you down. If that is the case, you will also find that your true friends are the ones who stand by your side and walk this journey with you.

Stigma Associated with Mental Health

In its simplest terms, stigma is when someone negatively views you because you have a distinguishing characteristic or personal trait that may be a disadvantage. Unfortunately, negative attitudes and beliefs toward people with mental health conditions are too common, but these attitudes' premise often comes from ignorance.

In my darkest moments before and after I attempted suicide, I had lost my purpose and felt alone. Those feelings were, in part, made worse for me because I have never been a person who shared their feelings and talked openly about what was happening in my life.

Sure, I talked to family and friends, but what I shared with them was what they wanted to hear, not what I felt. How could I possibly reveal to anyone that I believed I was a failure, that no matter what I did, it would never be good enough, that my father was right when he told my mother I would never amount to anything?

So when things turned upside down for me and our business, all these negative thoughts were reinforced, and the one thing I didn't need was a throwaway comment from the woman I loved that made me feel like an absolute failure.

Under the care of a psychologist, playing the game "tell them what they wanted to hear" and mixing with all of our friends and family, it quickly became apparent that I was viewed very differently due to my attempted suicide.

One of my closest friends and someone I thought I could rely on didn't know how to engage with me. Instead, he avoided me altogether, reinforcing my negative thoughts.

The funny thing about this situation was that I was happy because the last thing I wanted to do was pretend everything was normal and talk with these people. Over time, as I grew stronger, I realised the stigma still existed in our social and business engagements and interactions. My family didn't know how to help me navigate these challenging times, while everyone in the church took a step backwards or at least that's what it felt like.

Importantly, I realised that I was ashamed of what I did, and that feeling was as strong if not more robust than any stigma other people associated with my actions.

To put it into perspective, approximately 280 million, or 6% of people, suffer from depression, so don't think less of yourself because you are one of them.

Find someone who will listen and not judge who is a true friend because, at times like this, you discover your real friends.

Medication

While medication, from my perspective, is not an ideal solution, you need to understand that it will help and should only be used temporarily.

Some of the most commonly used include Selective serotonin reuptake inhibitors (SSRIs), such as citalopram (Celexa), escitalopram oxalate (Lexapro), fluoxetine (Prozac), fluvoxamine (Luvox), paroxetine HRI (Paxil), and sertraline (Zoloft).

SSRIs work by increasing serotonin levels in the brain.

Serotonin is a neurotransmitter (a messenger chemical that carries signals between nerve cells in the brain). It's thought to influence mood, emotion, and sleep.

After carrying a message, serotonin is usually reabsorbed by the nerve cells (known as "reuptake"). SSRIs work by blocking ("inhibiting") reuptake, meaning more serotonin is available to pass further messages between nearby nerve cells.

It would be too simplistic to say that low serotonin levels cause depression and mental health conditions. Still, a rise in serotonin levels can improve symptoms and make people more responsive to other types of treatment, such as CBT.

In any case, your doctor will prescribe the proper medication for you. You need to know that this treatment method should be temporary, and the depression returns should be restarted if stopped.

Psychological Theories

In psychology, six main theories provide the foundation for any therapy.

The Behaviorist Theory

Behaviour theory focuses on stimulus-response behaviours. According to this theory, all behaviours are learnt through environmental interactions.

The behaviourist theory in professional settings refers to the environment as stimuli, and the person's behaviour is a response.

The Psychodynamic Theory

The psychodynamic theory of psychology helps people look at their subconscious minds. Sigmund Freud believed everyone's subconscious contains an ID, ego, and superego. Each component includes subcomponents and plays its role in psychodynamic psychology.

The Humanistic Theory

The humanistic psychology theory primarily regards the individual's humanity and the different factors contributing to their feelings, actions, and self-image. To be precise, humanism states that each is unique in its own way and capable of change if it so chooses. The humanistic theory asserts that everyone bears responsibility for being happy and properly functional in the world.

The Cognitive Theory

The cognitive psychology theory asserts that human behaviours begin with a person's mindset. The cognitive approach primarily focuses on humans' attention, memory, and perception.

Biological Theory

The biological theory was primarily brought into inception via the studies of biologist and scientist Charles Darwin. The biological theory asserts that most behaviours are inherited and shaped by adaptation to one's external environment. According to this psychological theory, genes, DNA, and other hereditary factors impact human behaviour.

Getting Help

Mental health is the overall wellness of regulating your feelings and behaviours. Sometimes, people experience a significant disturbance in this cognitive functioning. A mental disorder may be present when patterns or changes in thinking, feeling, or behaving cause distress or disrupt a person's function. A mental health disorder may affect how well you:

- Marked personality changes, eating or sleeping patterns
- An inability to cope with problems or daily activities
- The feeling of disconnection or withdrawal from normal activities
- Unusual or "magical" thinking
- Excessive anxiety
- Prolonged sadness, depression or apathy

Mental Health Professionals

Everybody sometimes feels down, sad, frustrated, stressed or anxious, but it's important to recognise when a mood or behavioural change has become more than a temporary thing.

Only a trained health professional can diagnose someone with a mental health condition or disorder.

The best place to start is a trusted General Practitioner (GP).

When booking an appointment with your GP, ensure you book a more extended consultation to allow for discussion about how you are feeling and what concerns you have about your feelings. You don't have to tell anyone what it is for when booking, but I encouraged you to be as open as possible with your GP during the consultation so they have as much information as possible to help you.

If you are uncomfortable making an appointment, I suggest contacting one of the free help services.

Beyond Blue provides information and support to help everyone in Australia achieve their best possible mental health, regardless of age or where they live.

Summary

There is no quick solution when it comes to mental health. Instead, there is loneliness, doubt, fear, and anxiety. Being alone is not the answer; being in the company of others is unhelpful; you feel judged, angry, and despair, and the only solution seems to be ending the pain.

From my perspective, I wanted the people who pushed me to the edge to feel the pain; I wanted them to feel responsible for the actions I would take. Finally, the people I thought would understand, the friends I counted as closest, were unable or unwilling to help, and I felt like a leper, even though that was not the case.

I came to learn that the people I loved, I hurt, and the people I thought would understand didn't know what to say or how to approach me or help, so they avoided me, or at least that's how I felt.

The family will always turn up and be there for you, and my family did just that. I don't know what I would have done had I not seen them as my true north.

So, if you find yourself in this challenging and lonely space, don't try overthinking it; actions have consequences, and while they are challenging to overcome, you must trust that you are not alone.

"Mental health problems don't define who you are. They are something you experience. You walk in the rain and you feel the rain, but, importantly, YOU ARE NOT THE RAIN."

– Matt Haig

Chapter 14
Stress Management

We all deal with different levels of stress daily. Sometimes, that stress comes from the pressure of being unable to finish what you need within the time allotted; others, when the stress comes from losing something, you had every reason to believe it would be yours forever.

My greatest challenge with stress came from a critical health condition that resulted from acute nerve pain, my inability to cope with that pain, and the pressure it placed on my family. The compound effect and the financial strain of a mounting credit card debt brought me to stress levels I never thought possible.

Then, on that fateful day, nine words spoken in anger by my wife took me to the edge and to the point where I felt there was no other option but to take my own life.

I was angry with Jacqui, I was mad at myself, and I was furious with God. I remember driving around repeating those nine words as I contemplated how to end my life. In that stressed-out state, I failed to recognise the damage I was about to do to my wife and children. I certainly did not contemplate the effect my attempted suicide would have on them.

It has taken me years to repair the relationships with my daughters, and I am sure Jacqui still has moments of regret and disappointment. I know a day will come when the time is right when we will sit down and open up to each other.

From my perspective, I never wanted to talk about how I was feeling and when the psychologists tried to pry open my hidden vault of thoughts, I just gave them enough to satisfy but never the whole truth. Little alone, open up and talk to someone about what happened. I am not sure I even know the entire truth.

All I know is I just wanted it to stop, stop thinking, stop repeating those words, stop reliving the events, to have it stop.

Stress can take several forms, influence our thoughts and actions, and affect our lives. Following is an outline of the various types of stress.

Types of Stress

Stress is our built-in response to danger, the fight or flight fleeing. The threat may be real or imagined, immediate or far away when the hairs on your neck stand up. We know something isn't right.

According to the American Psychological Association, the three types of stress, acute stress, episodic acute stress, and chronic stress, all make us feel out of sorts, but chronic stress is often ignored.

Chronic stress: The grinding pressure wears us down over the years, and its origins come from serious life problems that may be beyond our control.

The demands are unrelenting, and you don't know when they will stop.

If you had a traumatic childhood, you might experience life as chronically stressful even when the surface appears OK.

Whether the cause lies in your mindset or difficult circumstances, many people stop fighting for change and begin accommodating chronic stress.

Episodic acute stress: Some people experience these mini-crises regularly and live in constant tension. They take on too much or are overburdened by life, resulting in increased tension and continuous anger.

You might need more time getting physical exercise while thinking through your issues.

Over time, a pattern of episodic acute stress can wear away in your relationships and work. That risk is greater with unhealthy coping strategies like binge drinking, overeating, or clinging to bad relationships. If poorly managed, episodic acute stress can contribute to serious illnesses like obesity, heart disease or clinical depression.

Acute Stress: You know the feeling when you're behind on a seemingly all-important deadline, and family issues and problems demand time you don't have to spare. When your heart races, your blood pressure rises, and you reach that point where you know what to do.

You become irritable, anxious, and sad and have headaches, back pain, and gut problems. These may appear for a short time and subside when the stress eases.

Our minds extend acute stress. A recent argument may replay in your mind, keeping you up at night. Or you might keep worrying about the future, a deadline ahead. Regardless of what type of stress you find yourself experiencing, you need to reach out for help, and the first place to start is with your local GP.

Effects of Stress on the Body

When your body senses danger, it releases stress hormones that cause short-term physical changes. These changes help you stay focused and alert until things are under control. However, if stress is constant and these changes persist, they can lead to severe problems in the long term, which may include the following:

- Aches and pains
- Chest pain or a feeling like your heart is racing
- Exhaustion or trouble sleeping
- Headaches, dizziness or shaking
- High blood pressure
- Muscle tension or jaw clenching
- Stomach or digestive problems
- Trouble having sex

Stress Management

Start with some straightforward changes, such as going to bed and getting up one hour earlier every day; that's right, Sundays included. Eliminate screen time and hot drinks before bed; eat 100 grams of protein thirty minutes before retiring.

A good night's sleep will be the second most crucial component of any stress management program.

Doctors don't know why, but people who exercise more tend to get better deep sleep, which helps renew the brain and body. Rest must balance the three levels: REM, Light, and Deep Sleep.

Exercise also seems to help mood by stimulating your body to release hormones like endorphins and endocannabinoids that help block pain, improve sleep, and sedate you. Endocannabinoids may be responsible for the euphoric feeling, or "runner's high", some people report after long runs.

People who exercise also tend to feel less anxious and more positive about themselves. When your body feels good, your mind often follows.

Exercises that will help are:

- Walking
- Running
- Swimming
- Dancing
- Cycling
- Aerobics
- Bike instead of driving to the store
- Use the stairs instead of the elevator
- Park your car as far as you can from the door
- Hand-wash your car
- Clean your house
- Walk on your lunch break

Diet

A healthy diet can lessen the effects of stress, build up your immune system, level your mood, and lower your blood pressure. Eliminating junk food, foods and drinks high in sugar from your diet can also help relieve stress.

To stay healthy and on an even keel, look for complex carbohydrates, lean proteins, and fatty acids in fish, meat, eggs, and nuts.

Antioxidants help, too. They protect your cells against damage that chronic stress can cause. You can find them in foods like beans, fruits, berries, vegetables, and spices like ginger.

Scientists have pinpointed some nutrients that help lessen the effects of stress on the body and mind. Be sure to get these as part of a balanced diet:

- Essential Vitamins
- Phytonutrient Diary Supplements
- Vitamin C
- Vitamin D

- Magnesium
- Omega-3 Fatty Acids

Relaxation Techniques

Yoga is an excellent form of exercise, but it can also be used as a meditation. There are many types of yoga, and the ones that focus on slow movement, stretching, and deep breathing are best for lowering your anxiety and stress.

Meditation: It has been around for over five thousand years for a reason. Meditation works well for many people and has many benefits. It can lower stress, anxiety, and chronic pain and improve sleep, energy, and mood.

Behaviour

How you respond to people directly impacts your stress levels. Manage your response with these tips:

- Try not to overcommit yourself
- Share the responsibility
- Count to 10 before you respond
- Walk away from a heated situation

Summary

Stress and how your body handles it can severely affect your health if neglected.

Effective stress management helps you break the hold stress has on your life, making you happier, healthier, and more productive. The ultimate goal is a balanced life, with time for work, relationships, relaxation, fun and the resilience to hold up under pressure and meet challenges head-on. But stress management is not one-size-fits-all. That's why it's essential to experiment and find out what works best for you.

Stress is not a physical object. It's a condition we allow to control how we feel and act; consequently, it can be turned down or off. We need to find the trigger that starts it in the first instance.

Waiting to deliver a presentation to an audience raises my stress levels. I am rarely stressed while preparing my materials, and once I have started delivery, all that stress fades away.

Looking at what is happening inside my head while waiting to start a presentation, I conclude that my head is full of last-minute doubts about the content. Have I included all the suitable materials and made all the correct assumptions, and will my audience understand my points and conclusions in my presentation?

My identity, belief system, and knowledge are the factors that unquestionably put me ahead of the game; I don't need to think about the what-ifs and the what-for because how I approach putting my presentations together far exceeds all expectations.

My identity, belief system and habits create an environment where all my presentations are made attractive, easy and satisfying, and as such, I know how to overcome that stress.

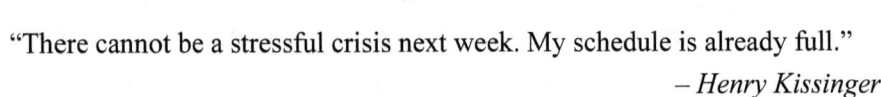

"There cannot be a stressful crisis next week. My schedule is already full."

– Henry Kissinger

Chapter 15
Environmental Health

Ecosystems

Like you and me, our ecosystem, known as Earth, is subject to change, and if ignored, the risk to its environmental health increases. The rising global average temperature is associated with widespread changes in weather patterns, such as heat waves. Large storms will likely become more frequent or intense with human-induced climate change.

More frequent and intense extreme heat events can increase illnesses and deaths, especially among vulnerable populations and damage crops. At the same time, increased precipitation can replenish water supplies and support agriculture; severe storms can damage property, cause loss of life and population displacement, and temporarily disrupt essential services such as transportation, telecommunications, energy, and water supplies.

Globally, sea levels have risen by about twenty centimetres since 1880. It is projected to grow another four centimetres to two point four metres by 2100 due to added water from melting land ice and the expansion of seawater as it warms.

In the next several decades, storm surges, high tides, rising sea levels, and land subsidence will increase flooding in many regions. These rising sea levels will continue past 2100 because the oceans take longer to respond to warmer conditions at the Earth's surface. Therefore, ocean waters will continue to warm, and sea levels will continue to rise for centuries at rates equal to or higher than the current century.

Our ecosystem will continue to change, accelerated under the sheer weight of these pressures and a growing population. At the same time, the quality of the food we grow and harvest and the water we need to sustain life will decline.

Using fertilisers and organically modified food is testimony to the impact on our capacity to grow the food required to sustain our growing population.

The earth's ecosystem, by definition, includes all the plants, animals, and organisms interacting with each other and non-living environments such as the weather, dirt, sun, soil, climate, and atmosphere. In this ecosystem, each organism has its role to play.

Earth's environment involves both living organisms and non-living physical conditions. These two are inseparable but interrelated, where the living and biological components are linked together through nutrient cycles and energy flows.

Organisms in an ecosystem are usually well-balanced with each other and their environment. An ecosystem may be natural or artificial and be land or water-based, while artificial systems could include cropland, a garden, a park or an aquarium.

Introducing new environmental factors or new species can have disastrous results, eventually leading to the collapse of an ecosystem and the death of its native species.

Ecosystems can vary in size, but they are usually places like forests and small ponds.

Australia's Great Barrier Reef is an example of a large ecosystem, while a small ecosystem could be the back of a spider crab's shell, which provides a home for plants and other animals.

Ecosystems are often separated by geographical barriers such as deserts, mountains, oceans, lakes and rivers, and the whole earth can be seen as a single ecosystem.

The quality of our farmed crops has struggled under the strain of demand, and our solution has been to use fertilisers to replenish the earth, causing the crops to be artificially enhanced. The drip-drip of nutrients into the creeks, rivers, and lakes from the fertilisers running off farmland causes algae to grow. As the algae bloom and decay, they leach oxygen from the water, unlocking nutrients in the lake bed and accelerating more growth and oxygen depletion.

We know that the risk of ecosystems collapsing today is heightened by intense stresses from industry, farming, and fishing, which often act together with global warming.

We must carefully monitor the subtle changes in our ecosystem structure and function that form the early warning signs of growing potential ecosystem failure.

Genetically Modified Foods

The genetic makeup of plants and animals has been manipulated for countless generations. It includes traditional cross-breeding of selected plants and animals with the most desirable disease resistance, high yield, and good meat quality characteristics for breeding the next generation.

Techniques identify particular characteristics and transfer them between living organisms, making it possible to copy a specific gene from the cells of a plant, animal or microbe and insert the copy into the cells of another organism to give the desired characteristic.

Corn with a gene that makes it resistant to insect attack or soybeans with a modified fatty acid content makes the oil better suited for frying. At the same time, plants that require less water to grow have also been developed to be more suitable for changing climatic conditions. Foods derived from genetically modified organisms are called 'GM foods'.

While it is impossible to predict the changes a genetically engineered species would make to the environment, it is reasonable to assume that any new genetically modified (GM) species could cause an imbalance in the ecology of an ecosystem.

Today, approximately 90% of the corn, soybeans, and sugar beets on the market are GM. Genetically engineered crops produce higher yields, have a longer shelf life, and resist diseases and pests.

On balance, it is believed that GM foods may harm the human body. Consuming these genetically engineered foods is considered to cause diseases immune to antibiotics.

Going Green

Going green is about pursuing knowledge and practices that can lead to more environmentally friendly and ecologically responsible decisions and lifestyles, which can help protect our environment and sustain its natural resources for current and future generations.

Going green can reduce air pollution and environmental toxins that affect our body's immune system, fight infections, and expose us to diseases and fatal illnesses. Another advantage of going green is that it helps decrease the pollutants released into our environment.

Going green has several positive environmental side effects that contribute to cleaner water and air, preserving natural resources and reducing the impact of global warming.

- Reduced Pollution
- Fewer Greenhouse Gas Emissions
- Resource Conservation
- Less Waste
- Wildlife Preservation

In short, it won't reverse the damage we have caused to our ecosystem, but it may just slow the damage we are doing down enough to help it recover to some extent.

The health of our ecosystem is just as important as our health; choose to do nothing about it, and eventually, it will fail.

Summary

I want to believe the message has been received by the people we have elected to govern. Still, the reality is that these issues are just too complicated and potentially already irreversible. We live in a beautiful but highly complex world, but believing these issues are reversible is simply delusional.

At some stage in the future, we will understand the changes our politicians should have made, and we will regret not having listened to the scientists and elected the people willing to make tough decisions.

"One of the first conditions of happiness is that the link between man and nature shall not be broken."

– Leo Tolstoy

Chapter 16
Long Life or Quality Life

People are Living Longer

According to WHO, people worldwide live longer and expect to live into their sixties and beyond. Every country in the world is experiencing growth in both the size and the proportion of its older citizens. The share of the population aged sixty years and over will increase from 1 billion in 2020 to 1.4 billion. By 2030, one in six people will be sixty years or over. By 2050, the world's sixty years and older population will double (2.1 billion). The number of persons aged eighty or older is expected to triple between 2020 and 2050 to reach 426 million.

Low and middle-income countries are now experiencing the most significant change. This shift in the distribution of a country's population towards older ages—known as population ageing—started in high-income countries (for example, in Japan, 30% of the population is already over sixty years old). By 2050, two-thirds of the world's population over sixty will live in low- and middle-income countries.

The United Nations General Assembly declared 2021-2030 the Decade of Healthy Ageing and asked WHO to lead the implementation. The Decade of Healthy Ageing is a global collaboration bringing together governments, civil society, international agencies, professionals, academia, the media and the private sector for ten years of concerted, catalytic and collaborative action to foster longer and healthier lives.

The Decade builds on the WHO Global Strategy and Action Plan and the United Nations Madrid International Plan of Action on Ageing. It supports realising the United Nations Agenda 2030 on Sustainable Development and the Sustainable Development Goals.

The Decade of Healthy Ageing (2021-2030) seeks to reduce health inequities and improve the lives of older people, their families and communities through collective action in four areas: changing how we think, feel and act towards age and ageism; developing communities in ways that foster the abilities of older people; delivering person-centred integrated care and primary health services responsive to older people; and providing more senior people who need it with access to quality long-term care.

Unhealthy Aging

With increased longevity came chronic, degenerative diseases such as heart and cardiovascular disease and cancer associated with older age. Successful treatments for those conditions have resulted in our ability to live longer.

Advances in the development of new medicines have drastically increased the human lifespan. They will continue to do so, but it needs to be realised that this approach treats illnesses over prevents them while neglecting the need for lifestyle modification that can reverse some conditions but significantly extend the quality of life in older age.

Humans seem lazy, and taking pills is more manageable than exercising.

Medicine will not cure; it treats the symptoms, and I would not have lived for as long as I have had it not for those medications. Medications sustained my life when I was unwilling to do whatever was required to reclaim my health.

Managing the Aging Process

As we grow older, we experience an increasing number of significant life changes.

- Career
- Retirement
- Loss of loved ones
- Physical health
- Mental health
- Isolation

I know from my experience that having lost both parents, mother-in-law, father-in-law, stepfather, and several friends while seeing my physical health deteriorate to a point where my wife believed she would become a widow. Four cancer operations in 2022, and that fear lived deep in her heart, given three of our parents died of cancer and cancer claimed the life of my stepfather.

How we handle these challenges is one of the keys to healthy ageing. Change is something we have learnt to live with all our lives, but coping with those changes is progressively more challenging as we get older and more isolated.

By necessity, learning to adapt to change may require finding new things to do and enjoy, staying physically and socially active, and feeling connected to your community and loved ones. Being active and mixing your physical activity with different exercise programs like walking, swimming, yoga, polarities, or anything else that takes your fancy will involve you with other people in your community. Importantly, don't ever forget that your ability to remain intense and focused will increase your resilience. It will go a long way to improving the quality of your health.

Coupled with a better eating program, something more in tune with your age, weight, and health ambitions or goals will give you a strong focus.

Taking responsibility for my health in September 2020 and deciding I would not lie down and let my life end was a turning point. Setting myself a goal and a time frame allowed me to focus on what I wanted and how I would transform my health.

Finally, it is never too late to start reframing your belief system and how you think about health. Whatever you do physically and eat, you need to work on how you feel about yourself and the identity that defines you. You may want to consider returning to university or doing a TAFE college course to build a new skill or hobby. Get that balance right, and you will not only extend your life but also the quality of your life, living it to the maximum.

Summary

At the age of seventy-three and faced with all my health issues, I reached that point where I either had to lay down and accept whatever was going to happen or get up and make an effort to change my life. Instead of the recorded messages I left on my phone for my wife and children, I took two pictures of myself, measured my chest, hips, waist and weight and defined in words where I was at that moment, where I was going to be and how I was going to achieve these objectives. I explained who I had been, who I would become, and how to accomplish this task.

At that point, I also started recording short sixty-second videos, which I started posting on Instagram to create a chronicle of my health journey, which I had hoped would give my family confidence in me and my efforts to reclaim my health.

I started with simple walks before breakfast of around four kilometres, or five thousand steps, starting at 5:00 am every morning, seven days a week, and over a year, I increased this to an average of twelve kilometres, sixteen thousand five hundred steps. Peripheral Neuropathy (caused by type 2 diabetes) had made my legs numb from the waist down, creating balancing issues and intermittent severe nerve pain while walking. Still, I just needed to push through this if I was going to redefine the man I needed to be for my family.

Twelve months after starting this journey, I would frequently back up my morning walk with a second walk in the afternoon of a similar distance, while the longest distance I walked in one day was thirty-two kilometres. In addition to walking, I have included a hundred pushups, seventy-five chin-ups and two three-minute planks to increase my fitness levels.

Extensive daily exercise and losing 40 kilograms in weight have resulted in my blood sugars falling back into the normal range. At the same time, the effects of peripheral neuropathy, including numbness and nerve pain, have improved considerably. While it may take a further two years for the nerves to recover from the damage caused by sugar, I am committed to gaining normal feelings in my legs while the nerve pain, which has already decreased by 80%, will continue to improve.

I am not remarkable, but I have become determined and am committed to reclaiming my health by overcoming challenging medical conditions. Along the way, I have also come to believe that anyone with enough determination can do what I have done, regardless of age; it starts with one step and a commitment to change the habits that have condemned our health.

"The air we breathe, the water we drink, and the land we inhabit are not only critical elements in the quality of life we enjoy, they reflect the majesty of our Creator."

– Rick Perry

Chapter 17
Wellness

Wellness is often confused with terms such as health, well-being and happiness. While there are common elements, wellness is distinguished by not referring to a static state of being (i.e., being happy, in good health, or a state of well-being). Instead, wellness is associated with awareness and choices that lead to optimal holistic health and well-being.

DOSE (Dopamine, Oxytocin, Serotonin, Endorphins)

These four main brain chemicals, *dopamine, serotonin, oxytocin and endorphins,* all play a role in how you experience happiness.

Dopamine

The chemical messenger, dopamine, is linked to the body's reward, motivation, memory, and attention functions. It regulates body movements while creating feelings of pleasure and reward, which motivates you to repeat a specific behaviour. In contrast, low dopamine levels are linked to reduced motivation and decreased enthusiasm for things that excite most people.

Oxytocin

Oxytocin is a hormone the hypothalamus produces and is secreted by the pituitary gland. It is an important hormone that plays a crucial role in childbirth, helps with male reproduction, and is an essential chemical messenger that controls some human behaviours and social interactions. Oxytocin triggers the bond between a mother and an infant and may also play a role in recognition, sexual arousal, trust, and anxiety.

Oxytocin has been nicknamed "the love hormone" because levels increase when you hug or kiss a loved one.

Low oxytocin levels have been linked to autism and autistic spectrum disorders, a vital element of these disorders being poor social functioning. Low oxytocin has been linked to depressive symptoms and has been proposed as a treatment for depressive disorders.

Serotonin

The chemical serotonin has varying roles in the human body. It is often called the happy chemical because of its direct effect on well-being and happiness. It plays a vital role in regulating mood balance. Low serotonin levels have been linked to depression.

As the precursor for melatonin, it helps regulate the body's sleep-wake cycles and the internal clock. It is thought to play a role in appetite, emotions, and motor, cognitive, and autonomic functions.

To increase your body's serotonin levels naturally, try modifying your diet, exercising, and exposing yourself to light.

Endorphins

Endorphin combines two words, endogenous, meaning inside the body and morphine, a medication that relieves pain. This powerful chemical is your body's natural painkiller.

Endorphins are connected to the feeling of no pain aspect of aerobic exercise and are produced in larger quantities during high-intensity anaerobic cardio and strength training exercises.

Time Changes Everything

They say time heals everything, which is probably true with some elements of my health journey in that I am no longer type-2 diabetic, and I've been able to get my hypertension under control to some extent. Still a little further to go.

But the one thing we need help to change is our habits. A habit that slowly steals your health without you even being aware.

As I have said, your health is like the air in a tyre. When fully inflated, everything works perfectly, but a slow leak will not be noticed until it's almost too late. Damage at that point can be unrepairable, cause additional issues with rims (kidneys), suspension (diabetes), and finally, cause a blowout (heart attack).

Health is a choice, and unless you are prepared to change your habits and everyday things slowly stealing your health, you must be ready to accept the consequences.

Wellness Influence

In recent years, wellness has become universal among consumers and businesses. Within a relatively short time, wellness has emerged as a lifestyle value, driving interest in fitness, healthy eating, self-care, mindfulness, stress reduction, wellness vacations, healthy ageing, complementary medicine, holistic health and other wellness practices.

Doctors, chiropractors, physiotherapists, and even psychologists have established buses that share the same business premises and, where needed, provide their service to the same client base.

Consumer interest in all things related to wellness is becoming a selling point for all kinds of products and services, from medical to chiropractic to mental health, dietary vitamins and gym memberships.

Healthcare Insurance companies recognise that encouraging their customers to join gyms by providing membership rebates has reduced their general insurance claims.

The Global Wellness Institute estimated wellness to be a $4.5 trillion market in 2017. Its growth rate has consistently outpaced global GDP growth, posting positive gains even in years of global economic downturn. What accounts for the seemingly unstoppable growth of wellness and its proliferation throughout the economy? In recent decades, profound financial, technological, social, demographic and environmental changes have transformed every aspect of our lives—our homes and communities, food, work, shopping, education, friendship, leisure, travel, etc.—with both positive and negative impacts on our health and well-being.

The growth of wellness practices and businesses is fundamentally a consumer response to these developments, and this response is turning into a significant societal and economic force.

Maintaining Wellness

By focusing on four areas of your life, you can change your health from substandard and feeling "just OK" to improving your vitality, health and attitude, thus optimising your wellness to feeling great every day.

- Improve your diet.
- Make exercise a daily part of your life.
- Supplement with vitamins and minerals, the food you feed your body is deficient.
- Reduce Stress.

Summary

I am not exceptional; I am just a man in a deplorable situation. I chose to accept that situation and that my life would end or force myself to change my habits and lifestyle.

When you stand on the edge of a cliff, rocking back and forth, fighting to hold your balance, your thoughts and actions are consumed with that task and nothing else. You fail to see what is happening all around you or to understand how much the people you love are lost waiting and watching to see what will happen.

We owe them, I owed them more, and I was failing them as the father and husband I needed to be, the man I wanted to be, the example I needed to be; I was dying on all fronts. I had allowed my health to decline, and I had been unwilling to fight to maintain it; how had I allowed myself to be so close to death on so many occasions and not realise what changes I needed to make?

Wellness is not a gift. We should all desire and be prepared to fight to achieve, fight as hard as it takes to live longer and improve life's quality and enjoyment.

"So many people spend their health gaining wealth, and then have to spend their wealth to regain their health."

– A. J. Reb Materi

Chapter 18
Why Most Diets Don't Work

The weight loss industry is projected to exceed 477.9 million in Australia, $2.8 billion in the USA by 2022, and $15.130 billion globally by 2028.

Do Diets Work is the Big Question

There is no question that diets, if adhered to, are more than capable of helping people lose weight; I should know because I lost between 25-35 kilograms on several of them. The problem is that it was the same 25-35 kilograms I put back on after I stopped the diet.

My problem with weight is my lifestyle choices, eating habits and a complete lack of willpower. While changing those habits was part of the process associated with losing weight, the habit was suppressed while I focused on losing weight. They returned once I had reached the weight loss goal.

Statistics show that 80% to 95% of people on a diet regain the weight they've worked so hard to lose.

Fad diets that reduce or restrict your calorie intake will allow you to lose weight, but you know you won't stay on that restrictive diet for the rest of your life, so your weight will increase over time as your old habits reappear.

In instances where the diet is too restrictive, your body moves into survival mode and does everything possible to prevent starvation, including:

Produces higher levels of leptin or ghrelin hormones, which controls how full you feel or makes you hungrier. Directs glucose as fat storage in the belief that you are in starvation mode and will need the energy later, while yo-yo dieting negatively affects your metabolism.

Your diet doesn't matter; rebound weight gain occurs almost every time.

To maintain weight loss for good, you need to focus on these four areas:

Diet: How can you create a healthy, long-term, stick-with-it diet?

- Learn what's healthy—and what's not.
- Learn what foods your body does not convert to energy and use and eliminate them from your diet.
- Exercise every day
- Drink more filtered water
- Change the way you think about food
- Change the habits associated with what you eat and the exercise you perform.

Exercise: Walking is a great way to improve or maintain your overall health. Thirty minutes daily can increase cardiovascular fitness, strengthen bones, reduce excess body fat, and boost muscle power and endurance.

Stress: Stress causes some people to eat more, raising the stress hormone cortisol levels. If you have more cortisol, you have higher insulin and lower blood sugar levels.

Sleep: Get the right amount of quality sleep every night. To improve sleep quality, go to bed an hour earlier every night, get up one hour earlier, and spend that time walking. Recently, after having surgery to remove two skin cancers from my face and still in a lot of discomfort, I decided not to do my regular morning walk, but as usual, I rose at 5:00 am and weighed myself. I went back to bed and slept until 9:30, which is unusual.

Surprisingly, when I weighed myself again, I lost 600 grams. If four and a half hours of sleep allowed my body to burn 600 grams, maybe I should go back to bed and have another rest instead of walking twelve kilometres every morning before breakfast.

Jacqui and I have tried a good number of diets, and while they all worked in the sense of us being able to lose weight, none of them addressed the issues that allowed us to become overweight in the first instance.

They all focused on the correct principles associated with weight loss and the importance of reducing our reliance on sweet foods, lollies, chocolates, soft drinks, and all other products manufactured to attract and retain consumers as regular customers.

Listed below are some of the more popular or well-known programs.

Rapid Loss

In 2013, I entered a weight loss competition with Rapid Loss. In the following sixteen weeks, he lost 28 kilograms, dramatically changing my overall medical condition. In February 2014, I won first prize and walked away with a cheque for $30,000. I also received a further $6,000 over the following six months for maintaining my weight while still on the program.

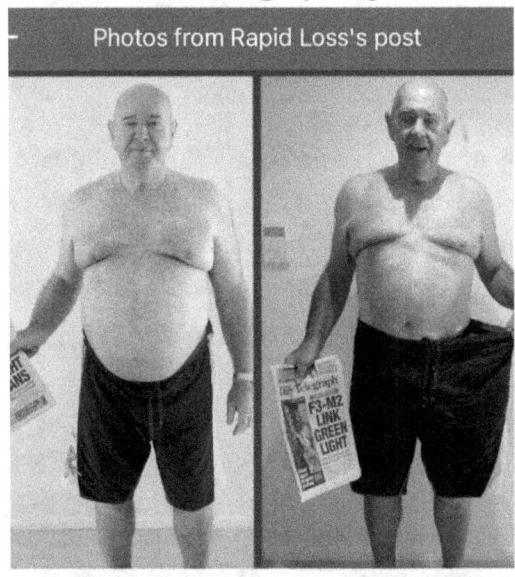

ROBERT LOST 27KG IN 16 WEEKS ON **RAPID LOSS**

I was also featured in the television commercial for Rapid Loss for several years until the company changed ownership.

When the monetary incentive to maintain my weight finished, I quickly lost interest in Rapid Loss as a dietary option. Rapid Loss is a meal replacement in a shake made of skim milk or water that forms a substantial part of my weight loss combined with regular exercise. While I continued physical activity for a little while, my old eating habits and weight rapidly returned.

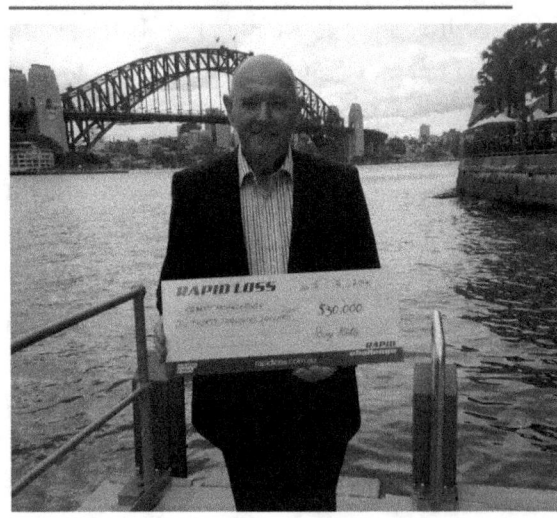

Fast forward to September 2020, and my weight had ballooned to 137.9 kilograms, and having survived a heart attack and a stroke, it was apparent some changes needed to be made.

Fit for Life

Harvey Diamond's Fit for Life is a diet plan that Harvey and Marilyn Diamond developed.

The diet formula works on the concept that eating a specific combination of food promotes good health. It also prohibits eating certain types of food altogether.

Jenny Craige

The Jenny Craig Rapid Results Max Weight Loss Plan consists of twenty-eight individually packaged food items (seven breakfasts, seven lunches, seven dinners and seven recharge bars). You will also receive a weekly coaching session with a Jenny Craig Coach on purchasing the plan.

Keto

The ketogenic (Keto) diet is a very low-carb, high-fat diet that shares many similarities with Atkins and other low-carb diets.

Lindora

Losing weight and keeping it off is about more than just counting calories. Lindora Clinic programs rooted in science offer a new approach to thinking about how you eat and live. This comprehensive lifestyle program teaches you to "Eat Better, Move More, and Stress Less". These core principles are the foundation of the program—and they work.

NOOM

Noom Weight is a weight loss program that helps you change your habits and mindset around food.

Rather than just focusing on what you should or shouldn't eat—like other weight loss programs—their psychology-based approach helps change your thoughts and feelings about eating.

Pritikin

The Pritikin Program was developed in the 1970s by Nathan Pritikin as a healthy lifestyle to aid weight loss and improve heart health. The diet emphasises eating unprocessed, low-fat, high-fib fibre foods and daily exercise.

Weight Watchers

The current WW (Weight Watchers) Freestyle plan is based on their SmartPoints system. Every food has an assigned number of points and you'll receive a daily budget of SmartPoints to use throughout the day.

Lindora Clinic

Losing weight and keeping it off is about more than just counting calories. Lindora Clinic programs offer a new approach to thinking about how you eat and live. Their program is a comprehensive lifestyle approach that teaches you how to "Eat Better, Move More, and Stress Less".

Why Don't Diets Work

The concept most diets are based on is setting a weight loss goal, and in that one word is the reason they fail and can succeed.

One That Does Work

With more than 15 million patient visits since 1971, Lindora Clinic has developed a deep understanding of the science of weight loss. With forty years of clinical research and experience, combined with a passion for continually improving and enhancing its program and protocols, Lindora Clinic is the gold standard in weight management.

Clinical physicians evaluate health risks such as heart disease, stroke, diabetes, abnormal cholesterol levels, insulin resistance, metabolic syndrome, and other preventable conditions and diseases associated with being overweight. The program aims to improve your health through weight loss, exercise, and other lifestyle changes.

One-on-one support during visits will help you stay focused and motivated. You'll learn how to activate your body's natural fat-burning system to burn stored fat for energy while protecting lean muscle.

Metabolic Adjustment will prepare you for successful weight maintenance at the end of your weight loss series. You begin another weight loss series if you have additional weight to lose because losing weight is only a partial victory when it comes down to it. Lasting long-term success is the ultimate goal.

Weight Loss Goal

A Goal is a final destination; it's the journey's end, nirvana, everything you want, and it relies on one thing to succeed, "willpower". The only problem with willpower is that we wouldn't be overweight in the first instance if it worked. So let's work around that word "Goal" and see where it takes us.

I believe for my age (seventy-four), my perfect weight is 96 kilograms, so I could set my weight loss goal at 96kg and know that with determination, I can reach the ideal weight, but can I maintain it and if I can, for how long can I maintain the weight. Alternatively, I know several habits have been challenging to break in my health journey, and I know how often I have not had the willpower to resist those temptations.

Realistically, does it matter that I failed to resist the temptation because there is always tomorrow and a new opportunity to exert willpower and change my habits?

The goal will get me there but not hold me there; willpower will work today and fail tomorrow, and habits are hard to change, so what's the answer?

Health Over Diet Works Every Time

The choice for me was straightforward: make changes that improve my health or face the consequences. With my kidneys rapidly approaching the point of failure and the inevitable need for regular dialysis treatments, the quality of my life and the burden I would place on my family was unthinkable.

How Did I Allow It to Get This Bad

No one by choice would let their life slowly slip away and not do whatever was required to change the outcome. Slowly, over thirty years, my health leaked from my body, and it became harder to fight back and easier to go with the flow.

When death is standing by our beds, waiting for that final breath, amazingly, at that point, we find the desire to fight, the strength to go another day, to hold or wait for that time, that critical date that person we want to see one last time, to say our final goodbyes to the people we love.

Health is "the state of being free from illness or injury".

I know what the word means, and I had health at one stage, but I don't remember when I started to lose it.

The problem is I don't think I ever owned it; I know I had it at one stage, but I never held it. Health was never part of my identity; it wasn't something that defined me, nor was it allowed to become a habit that described who I was and how others would identify me.

Instead, a thousand other habits consumed my life and filled it with pleasures and rewards, and I became a prisoner of the war they raged on my body and health.

What You Do is Who You Are

Who you are is part of the Identity Change you need to make to achieve the quality of health that will help you reach and maintain your ideal body weight. Remember, it's not a goal because once acquired, goals are the end of your destination, and your life will include many more years of quality health.

Don't get me wrong; I am not saying we should not have goals; instead, let's define them more at destination points based on continuous loop circling habits, goals and identity.

You affirm your true identity when you define yourself as a non-smoker rather than someone who has stopped smoking. Words, thoughts, affirmations, and originality reflect who you are, what you are trying to accomplish, and where you are going.

The concept of a continuous loop is simple; nothing in this world is static; it's constantly moving, as are the circumstances that shape our lives daily, so by continuously looping back through these three facets of your changing identity, you will always be in tune with who you are, who you need to become and who you will become and the habits you need to change as part of reaching the end of the loop.

Once your identity is firm in your mind, written clearly as part of your daily affirmations, your values, ethics, character, faith, and belief provide a continuous loop of improvement in self-belief.

As we approach the end of the book, I want to challenge you to ask yourself one straightforward question about your health: what do you like, what will drive you, and what will it take to be committed to achieving optimal health?

If you can't answer this, any quest to change has no real direction or future.

It's not about losing weight; it should never be about losing weight; it should always be how I live a life of the highest quality of health.

It's about being the person you want to be.

Summary

Health is a choice, and if health is what you want, then you need to start making changes to what you eat when you eat, what exercise you undertake, what identity you want to be associated with, what habit forms your identity and above all not become fixated with just losing weight.

Your identity relates to fundamental values that dictate our choices of who and what we value. For example, we can assume that a personal fitness trainer values fitness while a doctor values helping patients achieve good health.

Defining your identity allows you to identify the habits that align with that identity while changing your environment, making achieving those habits easier. When you change your environment, you have completed the circle to fuel the desired outcomes to achieve your health goals continuously.

Environment: what if I change my environment? I will grab a bin and work through the pantry, throwing out or giving away all the foods high in carbohydrates (sugar), eliminating them from my environment. So now your pantry is half empty, and the second part of changing your environment kicks into play; the weekly shopping list needs to be changed to avoid buying products similar to the one you have just thrown away.

With an emphasis on health, not weight loss, you need to define a list of the foods that will form part of your new identity and the environment that will support the change in eating habits you need to embrace. Develop new weekly menus that include fresh fruit and vegetables while eliminating processed foods and foods high in carbohydrates. Knowing what you will eat and ensuring you have an adequate supply of these essential foods is part of your changing environment.

Determining what you will do each day from a physical activity perspective is essential. It is necessary to ensure you have the right clothes and, very importantly, shoes for this lifestyle change. The best tip I can give you here is to buy two pairs of shoes so when the weather turns, and you finish your exercise routine with wet shoes, you will always have dry shoes the next day.

Hydration is essential with any physical exertion. Do not just drink water from the tap or buy bottled water; invest in a water purification system that filters and sanitises it simultaneously. Your body is a temple, and finding the health part of your new identity is selling yourself short if you don't respect that fact. While researching water for the book, I learned several critical points: drinking 600 milliliters of water before exercising will increase your body metabolism by 25%, which is a fantastic way to drop a few extra kilograms.

To become healthy and filled with energy, change the environment that supports the identity of the person you are.

Few people choose their identities. Instead, they inherit the values of their parents or the dominant cultures. In contrast, fulfilled people can live authentically to their values and achieve goals because those goals align with their identity.

Finally, the changes you want to make won't happen overnight, so I wanted to leave you with one sobering thought. Changing your identity, habits, and environment will have difficulties, but remember that anything is possible. You have just wanted it badly enough; preparing to accept it will take time.

In the book by Darren Hardy titled *The Compound Effect*, Darren talks about how you cannot improve something until you measure it. The incremental improvement over time of making a 1% daily improvement will blow your mind.

Thirty years ago, as a sales manager, I designed a method of measuring a salesperson's "micro selling skills", and I ran a statistical analysis of the compound improvement, making a slight 1% increase in a salesperson's selling skills would have on their conversion to sales ration. The analysis concluded that a 1% improvement in each of the five different selling skills over twelve months yielded a 35% increase in closed business.

Make health your priority and identity, but whatever you don't take for granted, as I did, you will only live to regret it.

"I tell people diets don't work. And I don't care what they say. I have tried them all."

– Sylvester Stallone

Chapter 19
Functional Medicine

Functional medicine recognises that illnesses do not occur in isolation and that symptoms and risk factors are associated with a person's health conditions and are governed by a person's clinical imbalances in the following biological systems, called nodes.

- Defence and Repair
- Energy
- Biotransformation and Elimination
- Transport
- Communication
- Structural Integrity
- Assimilation

Defence and Repair Node

Our immune system defends our body against what it perceives as foreign or a threat. When there is an imbalance, the result can be an overly active immune system or, the opposite, an immune system that cannot overcome infection.

Defence and Repair include chronic infections, allergic responses, food sensitivities and intolerances, and autoimmune disorders.

Factors influencing the Defence and Repair node include hormone imbalances, an inflammatory diet, infections, and exposure to substances unnatural to our environment, such as chemicals or heavy metal toxins.

Energy Node

In the human body, Energy is in the form of a chemical called adenosine triphosphate (ATP) and is produced in a critical part of the cell known as the mitochondria. For the cell to create ATP, it needs to break down simple sugar, fats, or proteins. The complex reactions that make ATP from these essential nutrients require co-factors or specific vitamins and minerals from a healthy diet.

Several toxins, including heavy metals, can slow the process of creating energy, while the mitochondria are susceptible to various factors that put oxidative stress on the cell. When there is more oxidative stress than the cell can handle, the cell can die.

Biotransformation and Elimination Node

Biotransformation and Elimination start from the day we are born and are essential for healthy, vibrant living. Chronic disease may occur due to disrupting the body's ability to eliminate the toxins it produces or from environmental exposures. Toxins can mimic hormones and nerve-signalling chemicals and wreak havoc on normal body functions.

Nutrient deficiencies, gut microbial imbalance, or genetic alterations can also affect the ability of the body to transform, break down, or eliminate waste.

Our industrialised culture, using plastics and other petrochemicals, herbicides, pesticides, pharmaceuticals, food additives, household cleaners, detergents, personal care products, and toxic metals, has greatly burdened what we have evolved to tolerate in our environment.

Transport Node

Transport applies to the conveyance of oxygen, nutrients and hormones in the bloodstream, electrons through the electron transport chain of the mitochondria, and the transport of messenger RNA into the cytoplasm (transcribed into a protein), molecules in the blood and cell membranes, fatty acids, essential minerals, and glucose.

Modifiable lifestyle factors of sleep, movement, nutrition, stress, and relationships should be evaluated for areas of need and corrective measures taken to improve balance within structural integrity and transport.

Communication Node

Communication refers to symptoms such as insomnia, fatigue, brain fog, abnormal menstrual periods, hair loss, cold intolerance, skin changes and weight gain. Poor libido, loss of genital sensitivity, and erectile difficulties can also be seen.

In the brain, the availability of neurotransmitters is dependent, in part, on the availability of the amino acids required to manufacture these nerve chemicals and normally functioning enzyme systems, which transform these building blocks into neurotransmitters and then help to break them down.

Structural Integrity Node

Structural integrity is necessary to repair and maintain the structure and tissue replication. Structural integrity in the intestines creates a selectively permeable barrier that allows nutrients to enter the bloodstream while excluding toxins and infections. When this barrier is disrupted, the result is a leaky gut. The blood-brain barrier in the skull is similar in function to the gut barrier. This structure prevents the free exchange of substances between the blood and brain tissue. Structural integrity can also refer to changes at the molecular level when transport proteins and receptors are altered in some way to affect their function.

Assimilation Node

Assimilation refers to the role of the digestive tract and its ability to break down and absorb nutrients, help regulate the excretion of water and electrolytes, and eliminate waste and toxins through the stool.

Increased gut permeability ("leaky gut") is one of the essential concepts in functional medicine and is the basis for most chronic diseases. To accomplish this goal, the digestive tract must maintain proper acidity in the stomach, have adequate amounts of digestive enzymes, and ensure the barrier that separates the inside of the intestines from the bloodstream is permeable only to nutrients needed for life. The gut's immune system and the population of microscopic organisms that inhabit the gut, known as the "microbiome", are critical to this process.

Finally, we also recognise the connectivity between the gut and the brain is a two-way street in which imbalances in the gut affect the brain, and the brain's activity affects the gut.

Summary

Functional medicine is an evidence-based, holistic approach to healthcare that embraces a shift from a traditional disease-focused approach towards a patient-centred approach.

When treating chronic disease, functional practitioners acknowledge a patient's biochemical individuality and involve patients in their healthcare plan as equal partners in planning their wellness.

Functional Medicine will look at lifestyle adjustments that focus on stress and physical inflammation being linked. Still, the link is somewhat mysterious, while conventional doctors avoid mentioning stress-induced inflammation.

However, functional doctors often suggest that patients reduce stress in their daily lives. Inflammation is the root cause of many medical conditions, and relieving stress may lead to less inflammation.

Research has confirmed that exercise therapy reduces depression and inflammation.

Examples of lifestyle changes include:
- Meditation, yoga, and spiritual enrichment
- Purifying the air or water in your house
- Adjustments to your social life, such as joining a local community group
- Spending time outdoors with your spouse or children each day
- A full night's sleep and
- Higher quality sleep
- Reduced alcohol consumption

Nutrition and Diet Counselling

From my perspective, changing my nutrition and diet has changed everything. It has allowed me to reduce what was sixteen prescription medications down to just four, allowed my kidneys to function for the first time in twenty years, cured my type 2 diabetes, lowered my blood pressure and allowed me to be pain-free.

Dietary supplements have significantly decreased my risk of disease while supporting me in recovering from cancer surgery.

Finally, I believe your choice of a local doctor and the relationship you build with that person are essential to finding suitable health and living a longer life.

Find a doctor who:

- Focuses on nutrition
- Opts for more natural treatments when available
- Emphasises partnership with the patient
- Spends significant time with each patient
- Has a higher education degree

Bibliography

Weight Loss Program Outline, "NOOM", Last Modified 13 January 2022
https://bit.ly/33uDrOe

Weight Loss Program Outline, "Diet Spotlight", Last Modified 13 January 2022
https://bit.ly/3qp5984

Weight Loss Program Outline, "KETO", Last Modified 13 January 2022
https://bit.ly/3zSaKqT

Weight Loss Program Outline, "Jenny Craige", Last Modified 13 January 2022
https://bit.ly/31TOiB9

Weight Loss Program Outline, "Fit For Life", Last Modified 13 January 2022
https://bit.ly/3qp5984

Weight Loss Program Outline, "Pritican", Last Modified 13 January 2022
https://bit.ly/3ri8WDL

Weight Loss Program Outline, "Rapid Loss", Last Modified 13 January 2022
https://bit.ly/3FlvCaT

Weight Loss Program Outline, "Weight Watchers", Last Modified 13 January 2022
https://bit.ly/3nm1eqU

Weight Loss Program Outline, "Lindora Clinic", Last Modified 19 April 2022
https://bit.ly/3uUhTWQ

Diets Don't Work, "BMJ", Last Modified 13 January 2022
https://bit.ly/3GiSjOp

Black Dog Institute, "Outline", Last Modified 13 January 2022
https://bit.ly/3rb7Pp7

Information on Heart Attacks, "Australian Heart Foundation", Last Modified 13 January 2022

https://bit.ly/33uII8u

Health Information, "Better Health", Last Modified 13 January 2022

https://bit.ly/31Rr0vw

Obesity, "WHO", Last Modified 13 January 2022

https://bit.ly/3rkTeI2

Overweight and Obesity, "Center for Disease Control and Prevention", Last Modified 19 August 2022

https://bit.ly/3A6AOiu

Sugar Intake, "WHO", Last Modified 13 January 2022

https://bit.ly/3rb9ETe

Nutrition Panel, "ANZ Food Standard Code", Last Modified 13 January 2022

https://bit.ly/33tTgVJ

Declines in Protein, "Science.Org", Last Modified 13 January 2022

https://bit.ly/3nlwBSw

Sydney Water Quality, "Australian Drinking Water Guidelines", Last Modified 13 January 2022

https://bit.ly/3niuWNq

Good Bad Cholesterol, "Heart Org", Last Modified 13 January 2022

https://bit.ly/3Gk3KFw

Coronary Heart Disease, "AIHW", Last Modified 13 January 2022

https://bit.ly/3K3CP34

Theories In Psychology, "Better Help", Last Modified 14 January 2022

https://bit.ly/3I3awzR

Getting Mental Health Help, "Beyond Blue", Last Modified 14 January 2022

https://bit.ly/3PzSRmE

Soil Degradation, "Department of Planning", Last Modified 26 January 2022

https://bit.ly/3IxHOaC

Index

2022

Prostate Cancer 58

7 Habits of Highly Effective

People 88

A balanced diet 168, 173
Acalculous gallbladder disease. 100
ACE 77
ACTN3 77
Acute Stress 203
Albumin 68
ALP... 67
ALT 68
Artificial sweeteners 171
AST... 68

Beyond Blue 200
Bicarbonate............................... 66
Biliary dyskinesia 101
Bilirubin..................................... 67
Biological Theory 199
BMI.. 187
BMI scale.................................. 133
Body Age................................... 188

Calcium 67, 157
Cancer of the gallbladder.......... 101
Carbohydrates................... 119, 168
Cardiovascular fitness 150
Central sleep apnoea.................. 45
Chloride............................... 66, 157
Cholecystitis 99
Cholesterol................................. 69
Chronic stress 203
CK 69
Coagulation and flocculation.... 165
Common Missing Nutrients in

Depleted Soil 158
Convenience Food.................... 172
Copper 157
CoQ10 181
Coronary Artery Calcium Score. 57
Coronary heart disease (CHD) ... 95
Corr Calcium 67
COVID-19 pandemic 194
Creatinine 66
Cryptosporidium...................... 163

Declining Nutrient Composition

.... 155
Depression 105

Diet 205
Dietary Fats 170
Dietary fibre 120
dopamine 147

Ecosystems 209
Effects of Stress on the Body ... 204
eFGR 65, 66
elements of sugar 118
endorphins 147
Episodic acute stress 203
Examples of Soil Degradation .. 154

Fasting
    One Hour, Two Hours 70
Fat 188
fat-soluble vitamins 156
fear and anger 135
Fear and Anger 37
Fibre 169
Fit for Life 229
Fluoride 157
From the Reservoir to the Tap .. 163

gallbladder disease 98
Gallstones 99
Genetically Modified Food 159
Genetically Modified Foods 211
GGT 68
Giardia 163
Globulin 69
Glucosamine 180

HbA1c 70
Healthy Weight Management ... 191
Hypertension 91

Insulin 69
Iodine 157
Iron 157

Jenny Craig 229

Keto 229
Kidney disease 108

Laparoscopic Radical
    Prostatectomy 61
LD 68
Lead poisoning 164
Leptorsirosis 23
Leptospirosis 23
Lindora Clinic 229, 230
lymph nodes 61

macrominerals 156
Magnesium 157, 181
Managing the Aging Process 215
Manganese 157
micronutrients 156
Micronutrients 156
Monounsaturated Fats 170
Monounsaturated fatty acids 121
Multi-vitamin 178
Muscle mass 189
Muscle Mass 189
My Identity 76

Nutrient pollution 167

Obesity 106
Obstructive sleep apnoea 45

Omega-3 178
Open Prostatectomy.................... 61
Osteoarthritis (OA).................... 103
Overweight and Obesity 189

pelvic floor................................. 61
Pelvic Floor Physiotherapy
    Training 63
People are Living Longer....... 214
peripheral nerves........................ 51
Peripheral Neuropathy.......... 51, 52
PET Scan 60
Phosphate.................................... 67
Phosphorus 157
Phytonutrients........................... 153
PI-RADS 5.................................. 59
Polyunsaturated fats.................. 121
Polyunsaturated Fats................ 170
Potassium........................... 66, 157
Primary hypertension................. 92
Pritikin 229
probiotic.................................... 177
prostate-specific antigen............. 56
Proteins 169
PSA... 69
PSA (prostate-specific antigen)..55
PSA (Prostate-Specific Antigen). 58

radical prostatectomy.................. 61
radioactive tracers...................... 60
Rapid Loss 228
Relaxation Techniques 206
Retrain Your Mind.................... 143
Robotic Prostatectomy 61

Saturated fats 120

Saturated Fats 170
sclerosing cholangitis 101
Secondary hypertension 92
Selenium................................... 157
Siberian Ginseng 179
signs of a stroke.......................... 54
Sodium 65, 157
Soil degradation........................ 152
Squamous Cell Carcinoma 138
Stage 3 Kidney Disease............. 24
Starch.. 119
Starches 169
Stigma Associated with Mental
    Health 196
Stress Management................... 204
stroke 95
Sugar... 170
Sugars 168
Sulphur.................................... 157
Symptoms of Sleep Apnoea 104

The Behaviorist Theory........... 198
The Cause of Declining Nutrient
    Composition 157
The Cognitive Theory 199
The Humanistic Theory........... 198
The Psychodynamic Theory..... 198
Total Protein.............................. 68
trace minerals 157
Triglycerides...................... 69, 94
Type-2 diabetes 94
Types of Stress 203

Understanding Blood Test Results
    65
Unhealthy Aging 215

Unsaturated fats 121
Unsaturated Fats 170
Urea 66
Uric Acid 67

Visceral fat............................... 188
Vitamin A 156
Vitamin B1 (thiamine)............ 156
Vitamin B12 (cobalamin) 156
Vitamin B2 (riboflavin) 156
Vitamin B3 (niacin) 156
Vitamin B5 (pantothenic acid)
    156
Vitamin B6 (pyridoxine) 156
Vitamin B7 (biotin)................. 156
Vitamin B9 (folate) 156
Vitamin C 180
Vitamin C (ascorbic acid) 156
vitamin D 178
Vitamin D 156

Vitamin E 156
Vitamin K................................. 156

Water Contamination and Required
    Treatments 164
Water Contaminations.............. 162
Water Ratios in Human Body... 165
Weight Watchers 230
Wellness 220
Wellness Influence 222
Willpower doesn't work 87

X chromosome 74

Y chromosomes......................... 74
Young Adults and Mental Health
    195

Zinc... 157

www.ingramcontent.com/pod-product-compliance
Lightning Source LLC
Chambersburg PA
CBHW070747310526
45791CB00028B/111